Computers for Nurses Made Easy

Computers for Nurses Made Easy

Karanbir Singh
Army Institute of Technology, Pune
E-mail: Karan_Kaos@hotmail.com

JAYPEE

JAYPEE BROTHERS MEDICAL PUBLISHERS
The Health Sciences Publisher
New Delhi | London

Jaypee Brothers Medical Publishers (P) Ltd

Headquarters
Jaypee Brothers Medical Publishers (P) Ltd
23/23-B, Ansari Road, Daryaganj
New Delhi 110 002, India
Phone: +91-11-23272143, +91-11-23272703
+91-11-23282021, +91-11-23245672
E-mail: jaypee@jaypeebrothers.com

Corporate Office
Jaypee Brothers Medical Publishers (P) Ltd.
4838/24, Ansari Road, Daryaganj
New Delhi 110 002, India
Phone: +91-11-43574357
Fax: +91-11-43574314
E-mail: jaypee@jaypeebrothers.com

Overseas Office
JP Medical Ltd
83 Victoria Street, London
SW1H 0HW (UK)
Phone: +44 20 3170 8910
E-mail: info@jpmedpub.com

EU GPSR Authorised Representative
Logos Europe, 9 rue Nicolas Poussin
17000, La Rochelle, France
Phone: +33 (0) 6 67 93 73 78
E-mail: Contact@logoseurope.eu

Website: www.jaypeebrothers.com
Website: www.jaypeedigital.com

Computers For Nurses Made Easy

First Edition: 2007, Reprint: **2026**

ISBN: 978-81-8448-047-4

Printed at: Samrat Offset Pvt. Ltd.

Preface

Professionalization for nurses involves the building of a strong foundation in nursing knowledge which is established, maintained, and constantly renewed through an ongoing program of research. With this knowledge the nursing profession can develop a theoretical basis for standards of practice which help clarify nursing roles and responsibilities

"The use of computers in health care is no longer a question for discussion and debate. Their application in nursing is a reality and is the need of the hour ...". With this statement, I propose to present a concise overview of the use of computers in nursing practice. The primary applications of computers are in the support of nursing documentation, patient care planning, and patient monitoring.

Nurses must spend a considerable amount of time documenting the care they are giving to their patients. In non-computerized environments, this involves writing the nursing notes in longhand. These notes report on the treatments, medications, procedures, diagnostic tests, and other components of the patient's health and activity over a certain period of time. In computerized environments, the documentation process can be automated through the use of standard reporting forms and checklists that allow the nurse to use various computer interface modalities to quickly enter the information concerning the patient. Menus, windows, pointing devices, or cursor keys can be used to select standard items from lists, while specific data (such as numeric values) can be entered via a keyboard. This automated documentation process not only saves time, but it also increases the accuracy of patient information and makes it more readily accessible for diagnostic or statistical analysis.

Computerized patient care planning can be implemented in a manner similar to the documentation process. Since standard lists of nursing diagnoses and interventions for particular patient problems have been prepared for almost all areas of nursing, it is not too great a leap to present these items via computer so that they can be selected and associated with particular patients.

Another big area of computer application in health care with major implications for nursing functions is patient monitoring. Dedicated computer controlled devices have been utilized for bedside monitoring of electro-cardiogram, heart and breathing rate, temperature, and various other vital physiological parameters for over 10 years. Presently these systems are becoming much more sophisticated and they are being integrated with the automated record keeping. In this way, the monitored status of the patient becomes associated with the nursing and medical records entered by members of the health care team. In addition to this, automatic posting of laboratory test results keeps the record current and further reduces nursing paper work (previously, lab reports would pile up on the desk until filed away in the patient's chart). In all, this automated and integrated patient record becomes a powerful tool for patient monitoring, record keeping, ongoing assessment, and evaluation.

In terms of more advanced applications for nursing practice, there are mentions of decision support systems in reference to possible applications of artificial intelligence. It is suggested that data collected by nurses in the process of assessing or monitoring the patient could be entered at bedside computer terminals and quickly processed by expert decision support systems to provide a more individualized set of possibilities for inclusion in the nursing care plan.

Informatics competencies include computer and information literacy skills as well as overall informatics activities. Computer literacy skills allow for the use of computer technology to accomplish tasks, such as using a word processor, database and spreadsheet or an application to document patient care or to communicate by e-mail. Information literacy is focused primarily on information access and evaluation. These skills enable an individual to recognize when information is needed and to locate, evaluate and use that information appropriately. Overall informatics activities may include using informatics applications designed for the practice of nursing.

It is hoped that this book proves to be useful in getting rid of any 'computer phobia' that the reader might have whatsoever. The language has been kept simple. Care has been taken not to overwhelm the reader with too much information in one sentence.

The chapters have been arranged in a fashion so as to make the understanding of the subject simple and progressive.

Lastly, in an effort of this kind, it is inevitable that some errors creep in. Necessary care has been taken to minimize the number of errors. Nevertheless, scope for further improvements remains and the author welcomes any suggestions to this end from teachers and students.

Karanbir Singh

Course Description

This course is designed to help students gain a basic understanding of the computers in order to utilize this in rendering effective nursing care in different settings.

General Objectives

Upon completion of this course, the students will be able to:

- Describe the basic Disk Operating System (DOS)
- Use computer for data processing
- Use computer for word processing and graphics
- Use computer in patient management system
- Use E-mail and the Internet

1. The contents of this book conform to the syllabi prescribed for the subject – 'Computers in Nursing'.
2. In addition to meeting this requirement, the book gives practical knowledge for the use of common computer programs in an easy form.
3. The book will therefore meet all theoretical as well as practical requirements.

Contents

1 **Introduction to Computers** **1**

2 **Operating Systems** **29**

3 **Introduction to Database** **53**

4 **Introduction to Windows** **70**

5 **Introduction to Word Processing and Microsoft Word** **85**

6 **Introduction to Microsoft Excel** **108**

7 **Introduction to Microsoft Powerpoint** **146**

8 **Introduction to Internet** **164**

Computer Jargon **183**

Index *189*

One

Introduction to Computers

Let us begin from scratch! COMPUTER...We all know what that word means: A small box which enables us to surf on the Internet, play extremely life-like games, listen to music and watch movies. Well, half a century ago the word referred to 'a person who performs computations'. At that time, there were no computers yet.

THE WORLD OF COMPUTERS

Have you used a computer recently? Chances are you have. If you have made a phone call, ridden in a car, watched a TV, played a video game you have used a computer. Even as you read this paper, keep in mind the words you are reading were put into type by a computer.

Here is a list of statements about computers. Decide whether each statement is **true** or **false**.

1. Computers are smarter than humans.
2. Computers have brains.
3. Some computers have feelings.
4. Computers can solve any problems.
5. You need to know a lot of science and math to use a computer.

If you decided that each statement is false, you are correct. Then what is a computer? What can it do? It is, basically, a machine that can handle large amounts of information and work with amazing speed. **A computer is built to do these four jobs:**

1. **Accept information:** You can put raw data into it. The information might be a collection of facts and figures or possibly a set of instructions to the computer telling it what to do.

2. **Store information:** It has a device called the memory (described later in this chapter) that holds the information as long as you want it to.
3. **Process the information:** This means it does something with the information. It might do an addition problem or compare and sort the information depending upon the users' wish.
4. **Give out the processed information:** It gives you the results of the processing which are, indeed, the results of the instructions given to the computer by the user.

Computers are conformed to follow instructions from humans. They can solve only the problems that people tell them to solve. Since people cannot solve every problem, neither can computers. To tell a computer what to do, you have to know what problem you want to solve and should have a plan for solving it.

Since computers can't do anything without instructions from a human, what makes them so special? They can do some things better than humans. Computers calculate faster than humans. They are more accurate than humans. Computer can also store vast amounts of information and they do not "forget" what they store. These kinds of qualities make computer wonderful tools to help people solve complex problems.

Hence, a computer is a device that accepts information and manipulates it for some result.

Computers can be confusing and it takes a little time before you gain confidence in using and understanding them. Just like a new TV or VCR, computers can be a bit cumbersome to figure out, but once you achieve a certain level of knowledge, these machines can become powerful allies.

Don't be afraid to tinker around on a computer. Like learning to drive or riding a bike, computing simply takes patience and practice!

COMPUTER BASICS

Let's try a simple approach....
A library is a big building, in this case we are visiting a random library. So a library when it is first built is simply a big empty building. Similarly, a computer is simply an empty metal box until you put the parts in.

Ok, a library needs someone to run it, a librarian ... A computer needs someone to run it, a CPU or processor chip.

A librarian needs a name, Betty, Nancy, Ramu, Shamu, Chimpu ... A computer "Chip" needs a name, 486, Celeron, Pentium I, Pentium II, Pentium III, Pentium IV, etc.

No matter what the librarian's name is, a librarian is the person that runs the library and makes all the decisions. No matter what the processor chips name, the chip is the part of the computer that runs the computer and makes all the decisions.

The faster the librarian in a library, the faster the work gets done. Similarly, the faster a processor chip, the faster the actions are performed.

The oldest and thus the slowest chip listed here is the 8086, then came the 286, 386, 486, etc. With each one being faster than the chip before it. Finally a new chip was invented that was even faster. It was named Penny. As in the Pentium I. Few years ago came the fastest chip available to home PC users called the Pentium IV... And right at this moment as you read this…there are people working to develop a faster processor still.

With librarians and processor chips, if you are waiting, faster is better. With that I want to mention that each chip is listed with a processing speed. As any child can tell you the bigger the number, the faster the computer. So if someone tells you that their librarian can stack 100 books an hour and your librarian can stack 200, then you know your librarian is faster.

So a computer that has a speed of 2.1 GHz (Giga Hertz), is slower than one with 3.2 GHz. The speed is referred to the processing speed or you can think of it is the "speed of thought" of your librarian.

COMPUTERS — HOW THEY WORK AND RELATED TERMS

Why is it important to know how computers work? Easy, if you don't, they will be hard to control. Computers were never built to control us even though that is how it appears. Their creation was just another tool to be used to benefit society. What can you do to learn more about computers? There is an easy answer. Just read and use computers more. They are not that hard and with time you too can become the master over this tool.

Computers, the ones we know have not been around for that long. The first home personal computer was not sold until **1977**. We have come a long way since then. Did you know that in **1983** there were approximately *2 million* personal computers in use in the United States? However, just 10 years later in **1993** the number had jumped to more than *90 million*.

Computers, today are small, fast, reliable and extremely useful. Back in 1977 that really was not the case. However, they both operated in basically the same way. They both receive data, stored data, processed data and then output data similar the way our own brain functions. Following are the ***4 functions*** that a computer performs:

A. **Memory**
B. **Processing**
C. **Input** and
D. **Output**.

MEMORY

Let's look at computer memory first. The function of storage in a computer comes in many different sizes, types and shapes. However, there are two basic categories: **short-term memory** and **long-term memory**. A typical computer contains numerous types of memory including **RAM**, **ROM**, **virtual**, **cache** and various long-term storage devices. Each type of computer memory serves a specific function and purpose.

The computer must be given instructions, in the form of software, which tells it exactly what to do. The instructions that the computer follows are stored in locations known as memory. For simplicity purposes think of memory in two categories:

1. The computer's **Internal memory** (e.g. microchips)
2. The computer's **External memory** (e.g. diskettes and hard drives).

Computer memory is measured in bytes (Refer to **Fig. 1.1**). A single byte is made up of a series of **1's** and **0's** normally traveling in pairs of eight. These eight 0's and 1's are the way the computer communicates and stores information. With each keystroke or character a **byte** of memory is used.

8 bits	=	1 byte
1024 bytes	=	1 kilobyte
1024 kilobytes	=	1 megabyte
1024 megabytes	=	1 gigabyte
1024 gigabytes	=	1 terabyte

Fig. 1.1: Measuring Bytes

The computer's internal memory which is composed of computer chips is divided into two types: RAM (random-access memory) and ROM (read-only memory).

ROM

ROM or **Read-Only Memory** is permanent, long-term, **nonvolatile** memory. Nonvolatile means is does not disappear when the computer is shut off. It also cannot be erased or changed in anyway. ROM's primary purpose is to store important instructions that the computer will reuse over and over such as what to do when the computer is turned on and how to control specific requests made by the computer.

ROM is permanent memory that cannot be changed or erased. This is why it is called Read-Only Memory.

RAM

RAM or **Random-Access Memory** unlike ROM works only when the computer is turned on. This memory is **vital** to the computer because it controls the **moment** by **moment processes** of the computer. The first thing that goes into RAM is the **OS (operating system)**, which in most cases is some version of Windows. Next, for the RAM is an application program that might be a game or the Internet browser, etc.

RAM's primary purpose is to temporarily store programs given to it by a programmer or operator of the computer. This type of memory is temporary because it is erased when the computer is turned off (powered down). In other words, all the information in RAM is erased when the computer is turned off. It is called random access because the processor can jump directly form one location to another in random order as the program is needed.

Multitasking has put more demand on RAM in the past few years. Multitasking is the *ability to run more than one* program at the same time. For instance, many people like to listen to music along with their word processing software. This means you need lots of RAM to hold both programs.

Other types of temporary-memory are **cache** (pronounced "cash") and **virtual memory**. Both of these types of memory supplement the computer's primary RAM and perform the same function as RAM.

Storage Devices

RAM and ROM may be very important parts of the computer; however, without storage devices like hard drives and disk drives your computer would not be near as useful.

DISK DRIVES

Let's go back to our library again...

We have a librarian and she has to put away the books. She needs someplace to store these ... there are several rooms in the building and so she gives each one a name so that she knows which room is which. Books simply sit in these rooms until someone wants to read them. If the books are put away neatly, saved and there is a power outage, when the power comes back on, the books are still where she put them.

Okay, the computer is basically a library where you store books. The books are called files, programs, etc. The computer librarian needs someplace to put your books. These storage areas are called disk drives.

Every computer has a main disk drive called your hard drive. It is normally called your "**C**" drive and is written like this C:\

Once you "Save" something to this drive, it is there whether you turn off the computer or not. When you are typing, things are in a temporary work area and can be lost unless you save them. So it is advisable to save them often!

Your main library is huge. It is rated in Megabytes (MB) or Gigabytes (GB). The bigger your hard drive the more storage space you have for (books) files, graphics, programs. If you start to run out of space though, old unneeded files (books) can be deleted (thrown away) to make room for new ones.

Your computer has one big Hard Drive "C" which is the main room of the library. But you need to have some way to store extra books that won't fit in your library or that you want to take to work with you. Think of these as the storage carts that a librarian uses. Without the carts it would be impossible for the librarian to transport all the files from one place to another and the building might explode if you kept to much information inside.

And the same is true of computers. We need a way to save some things to carry with us to share with friends at work or to keep as an emergency backup in case of a system failure.

This method of storage is referred to as a disk. Disks come in basically three different sizes. Diskettes (3.5 inches wide), CDs and DVDS (compact disks), Zip Drive Disks.

Diskettes hold a small amount of information (1.44 MB) and can be used to write information from the computer or to read information from the disk to be used inside the computer. These are also a good way to take your important files to an office computer, etc.

CDs (CDs or compact disks) can hold a huge amount of information. There are two types of write-able CDs: CD-RW and CD-R.

1. **CD-R**: These are very inexpensive disks that can only be written onto (burned) one time. Whatever is written onto them is permanent. Think of it as though the disk had been written on in ink.
2. **CD-RW**: The disks are more expensive, but you can write on them, erase them, write on them again, over and over. In other words, you can use them over and over again for different things. Think of these disks as having been written on in pencil. You can erase them and use them over again.

Either disk can be written (burned) using a CD Burner (CD writer) and so you can copy files, songs, etc. onto these disks to share with your friends, use them for storage, etc.

Zip Disks can hold a wealth of information. Many are now portable and can carry anywhere from 100 MB of data to 3-4 GB of data.

So, if you understand all a disk drive does is store information, then you understand disks.

The most common forms of storage devices found on computers are illustrated in Figure 1.2.

PROCESSING

If someone had to find the **brains** of the computer they would most certainly say it's the **microprocessor**. The computer chip that receives and carries out these instructions is called the processor. All computer systems, regardless of size or manufacturer, have processors (also referred to as central processing units or CPUs). The microprocessor is a chip, the size of a **postage stamp**. The processor is the one part of the computer that is most important to the computer. The microprocessor controls how data is sorted and directs the flow of data.

All computers do processing by following a series of instructions in a software program. The processor performs many different functions. It receives and temporarily stores instructions as well as the data to be processed. It moves and changes stored data. It does arithmetic calculations. It makes decisions of logic, such as determining if two numbers are equal. It directs the action of the input and output devices.

Floppy disk or floppy	A round plastic surface that is coated with magnetic film. They come in $3^1/_2''$ size. They hold about 720 to 1440 k of information. They are typically used to save, share and/or copy files. Floppy drives are given letters. Commonly the floppy is A, a 2nd floppy is B and the hard drive is C.
Hard disk (drive) or HD	A stack of round metal platters called disks encased in a metal air-tight shell. They commonly range in sizes from 20 to 100 gigabytes (1024 MB = 1GB). The hard drive's function is to store all the files and software the computer will ever use. Any file or software program used by RAM most likely will come from the disk drive.
CD-ROM (Compact disk, read-only memory)	CDs function much like hard drive in that they store large amounts of memory. What separates them is their mobility and optical storage technology. Their storage capacity is also very limited compared to hard drives. The can only hold up to approximately 700 MB of information. The other big difference is that you have to have a special drive to write to CD's. Otherwise they can only be read from.
DVD-ROM (Digital video disk, read-only memory)	DVDs are similar to CD in that they are written and read by laser. Hard drives use magnetic currents store data. However, CDs and DVDs use light (laser) to write and read data on a disk. These long and short pits are then stored or etched on the surface of the disk. They can only be read by laser technology. The new DVD technology increased the amount of memory a regular CD can hold. DVDs can range in sizes from 4.34 GB (1024 MB = 1GB) to 7.95 GB.

Fig. 1.2: Types of storage media

To a great extent a computer is defined by the power of its microprocessor. Chips with higher processing speed and more recent design offer the greatest performance and access to new technologies. Most microprocessors made for PCs are made by **Intel** or by companies that clone Intel chips, such as Advanced Micro Devices (**AMD**) and **Cyrix**.

INPUT

One of the best features of a computer is the ability to give the computer commands and feed it information. Without an input device this would not be possible. **A hardware device which enables the computer to accept data is called an input device.** The most common example of an input device is a keyboard and a mouse. Input devices can be built into the computer, like the keyboard in a laptop or it can be connected to the computer by a cable. There are lots of others such as: **trackballs**, **touch pads**, **touch screens**, **pens**, **joy sticks**, **scanners**, **bar code readers**, **video** and **digital cameras** and **microphones**. In addition, storage devices such as disk drives can serve as input devices.

OUTPUT

Input is important but equally important is the ability to read what the computer is doing. The computer output devices are used to serve the user. **A hardware device which reports the information in a form we can understand is called an output device**. The most common output device is the **monitor** or **screen**. However, most computer come with **speakers** and a **printer** which are excellent output devices. Storage devices such as **disk drives** and **diskettes** also serve as output devices when it is necessary to write new or updated data files to disk or tape.

EXPLORING COMPUTERS

Hardware and Software

Computers are made up of hardware and software. Hardware is the tangible, physical equipment that can be seen and touched. Examples of hardware are things such as the keyboard, printer, monitor and computer chips.

Software is the intangible instructions that tell the computer what to do. Software are things such as games, MS Word, etc. People who write software (instructions that tell the computer what to do) are called programmers.

Programmers write instructions or programs, to the computer so that it is able to execute a task or operate properly. A program can be defined as a series of detailed step-by-step instructions that tell the computer precisely what actions to perform.

Many people believe that computers can do just about anything and that their level of sophistication requires a genius to program and run them. In reality, computers are very simple devices that can perform only four basic functions. A computer can:

1. Store data and programs
2. Function unattended due to its ability to interpret and follow instructions it is provided
3. Do arithmetic calculations and
4. Perform logical comparisons.

What makes the computer such a powerful device, given only these four basic functions, is its tremendous speed, its accuracy and its ability to store vast volumes of data.

External or Auxiliary Storage

Nearly all general-purpose computers include the ability to connect to additional storage devices that hold data outside the memory of the computer. These additional storage devices are known as external or auxiliary storage. External storage devices are on-line to the computer; that is, they are connected directly to the computer. They are, therefore, under the control of the processor and can be used at all times. The most common form of external storage is a disk drive. Other forms of external storage include hard drives and CD-ROM drives.

The disk drive records data in a method similar to that used by a cassette tape recorder. The information is actually magnetically encoded into the floppy disk. External storage is used to hold computer programs so they may be read into the computer's random-access memory (RAM) when they are needed. Large amounts of data may also be stored on external storage. Remember from an earlier section that data is stored in RAM is temporary. Therefore, any data that is needed to be kept for future use is usually recorded on a magnetic disk before the computer is powered down.

Microchips

Scientists all over the world are trying to overcome the physical limits of chip design technology that began less than three decades ago. Each country is rushing to be the first to develop micro-computer chips that contain one billion transistors.

Transistor technology preceded chip technology. Transistors were smaller, more efficient and more reliable than their predecessors the vacuum tubes. The major limitation of transistors was in their limited number of interconnections. In other words, because of the sophisticated circuitry of computers, an enormous number of connections between transistors were required. Unlike the number of transistor connections needed in a radio, the number of transistor connections in computers extends into the millions. Chip technology solved the interconnections problem by placing several transistors on a tiny silicon surface. Thus, computer power and storage capabilities expanded dramatically.

The number of transistors which can be placed on a chip has increased from fewer than ten in the early chips to thousands in the chips used today. Chip technology has enabled the chip's capacity to double every year since its creation until just a few years ago. However, today's chip designers have run into a problem concerning the physical limitations of a single chip; therefore, the interconnections problem of the transistor technology has resurfaced.

THE COMPUTER'S WORLD

To help you understand how the computer works, imagine that each character is represented inside the computer by a series of electronic switches. In many ways, these electronic switches can be compared to the light switches in our home. A light switch can be in only one of two states: on or off. The circuits inside the computer can be thought of in much the same way as the light switches. The electronic switches can be either on or off. Since on and off represent only two conditions, it is impossible to directly store numbers or letters. Instead, they are converted into binary numbers. Binary means "consisting of two things", so a binary number is made by using only two digits, 0 and 1. Our and much of the world's number system is based on the 10 system but the computer's system is based on the binary system. Therefore the binary number system is the only coding system the computer actually understands.

But, in order to actually understand and then appreciate the present state of the world of COMPUTERS, we must know how it all started...

EVOLUTION OF COMPUTERS

Calculating machines capable of performing the elementary operations of arithmetic (addition, subtraction multiplication and devision) appeared in the 16th century. These were clever mechanical devices constructed from gears, levers and the like. The French philosopher Blaise Pascal invented a mechanical calculator that could add and subtract decimal numbers. Decimal numbers were engraved on the counter wheels much like those in a car's odometer or in the counter in a petrol delevering machine. In Germany, Gottfriend Leibniz extented Pascal's design to one that could also perform multiplication and division.

The evolution of the computers can be explained mainly on their five generations, as follows:

GENERATIONS OF COMPUTERS

The history of computer development is often referred to in reference to the different generations of computing devices. A generation refers to the state of improvement in the development of a product. This term is also used in the different advancements of computer technology. Each generation of computer is characterized by a major technological development that fundamentally changed the way computers operate, resulting in increasingly smaller, cheaper, more powerful and more efficient and reliable devices. As a result of the **miniaturization**, **speed**, **power** and **memory** of computers have proportionally increased. New discoveries are constantly being developed that affect the way we live, work and play.

Read about each generation and the developments that led to the current devices that we use today.

The Zeroth Generation: Mechanical Computers

In the 19th century Chalrles Babbage designed the first computer to perform multistep operations automatically, that is, without a human involement at every step. It was entirely mechanical in nature. He called it – The Difference Engine.

It was designed to compute and print mathematical tables automatically. The Difference Engine only performed one arithmatic operation — addition. However, using the Method of Finite Difference included in the Difference Engine, it can calculate many complex and useful functions by means of addition alone. The most interesting feature of the difference engine was its output method: it punched its results onto a copper engraver's plate with a steel die.

The ELECTRONIC ERA began...

The first electric computer apperared in the 1940s. Since then development has reached an enormous rate. The Second World War brought changes in every walk of life. During the war precise machines were needed for ballistic calculations and hence the need of 'something' was felt.

The First Generation (1946-1958)
The Vacuum Tube Years

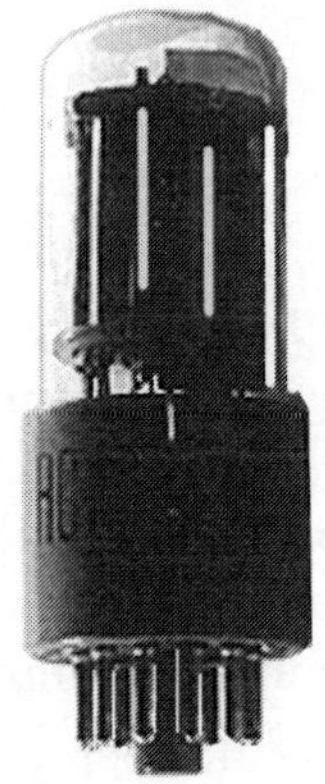

Fig. 1.3: A vacuum tube

The first computers used vacuum tubes (**Fig. 1.3**) for circuitry and magnetic drums for memory and were often enormous, taking up entire rooms. They were very expensive to operate and in addition to using a great deal of electricity, generated a lot of heat, which was often the cause of malfunctions. First generation computers relied on machine language to perform operations and they could only solve one problem at a time. Input was based on punched cards and paper tape and output was displayed on printouts. The first generation computers were huge, slow, expensive and often undependable.

The vacuum tube was an extremely important step in the advancement of computers. Vacuum tubes were invented the same time the **light bulb** was invented by Thomas Edison and worked very similar to light bulbs. Its purpose was to act like an ***amplifier*** and a ***switch***. Without any moving parts, vacuum tubes could take very weak signals and make the signal stronger (***amplify it***). Vacuum tubes could also stop and start the flow of electricity instantly (***switch***).

In **1946, based upon the above mentioned properties,** two Americans, Presper **Eckert** and John **Mauchly** built the **ENIAC** (Electronic Number Integrator and Calculator) which used vacuum tubes instead of the mechanical switches of the **Mark I**. The ENIAC used thousands of vacuum tubes, which took up a lot of space and gave off a great deal of heat just like light bulbs do. The ENIAC led to other vacuum tube type computers like the **EDVAC** (Electronic Discrete Variable Automatic Computer) and the **UNIVAC I** (UNIVersal Automatic Computer).

The UNIVAC (Universal Automatic Calculator) and ENIAC (Electronic Numerical Integrator and Calculator) computers are examples of first-generation computing devices. The UNIVAC was the first commercial computer delivered to a business client, the US Census Bureau in 1951.

ENIAC was the first generation of today's modern computers. But, by today's standards for electronic computers the ENIAC was a grotesque monster. Its thirty separate units, plus power supply and forced-air cooling, weighed over thirty tons. Its 19,000 vacuum tubes, 1,500 relays and hundreds of thousands of resistors, capacitors and inductors consumed almost 200 kilowatts of electrical power.

ENIAC could discriminate the sign of a number, compare quantities for equality, add, subtract, multiply, divide and extract square roots. ENIAC stored a maximum of twenty 10-digit decimal numbers. Its accumulators combined the functions of an adding machine and storage unit. No central memory unit existed, storage was localized within the functioning units of the computer.

The primary aim of the designers was to achieve speed by making ENIAC as all-electronic as possible. The only mechanical elements in the final product were actually external to the calculator itself. These were an IBM card reader for input, a card punch for output and the 1,500 associated relays.

It is interesting, that the creation of the first real computers is linked to a Hungarian scientist, Neumann János. After graduating at the University of Budapest he was invited to the University of Priceton in 1930. Three years later he became one of the six mathematics professors at the Institute of Advanced Studies (IAS). He worked out the basic concepts of modern computers.

The ENIAC gave off so much **heat** that they had to be cooled by gigantic air conditioners. However, even with these huge coolers, vacuum tubes still overheated regularly. It was time for something new.

The Second Generation/(1959-1964)
The Era of the Transistors

Just like the evolution of televisions, radios and amplifiers during this time revolved around the shift from vacuum tube to transistor, so did computers. The use of transistors (Refer to **Fig. 1.4**) allowed radios, TVs, amplifiers and computers to become much smaller, faster, less energy draining, etc.

The transistor computer did not last as long as the vacuum tube computer lasted, but it was no less important in the advancement of computer technology. In 1947 three scientists, **John Bardeen**, **William Shockley** and **Walter Brattain** working at **AT and T's Bell Labs** invented what would replace the vacuum tube forever. This invention was the **transistor** which functions like a vacuum tube in that it can be used to relay and switch electronic signals.

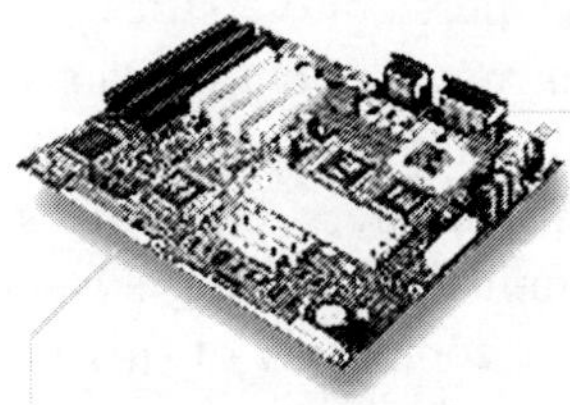

Fig. 1.4: Transistor

There were obvious differences between the transistor and the vacuum tube. The transistor was faster, more reliable, smaller and much cheaper to build than a vacuum tube. One transistor replaced the equivalent of *40 vacuum tubes*. These transistors were made of solid material, some of which is **silicon**, an abundant element (second only to oxygen) found in beach sand and glass. Therefore they were very cheap to produce. Transistors were found to **conduct electricity faster** and **better** than vacuum tubes. They were also much **smaller** and gave off virtually **no heat** compared to vacuum tubes. Their use marked a new beginning for the computer. Without this invention, space travel in the 1960s would not have been possible. However, a new invention would even further advance our ability to use computers.

Transistors replaced vacuum tubes and ushered in the second generation of computers. The transistor was invented in 1947 but did not see widespread use in computers until the late 50s. The transistor was far superior to the vacuum tube, allowing computers to become smaller, faster, cheaper, more energy-efficient and more reliable than their first-generation predecessors. Though the transistor still generated a great deal of heat that subjected the computer to damage, it was a vast improvement over the vacuum tube. Second generation computers still relied on punched cards for input and printouts for output.

Second generation computers moved from cryptic binary (0s and 1s) machine language to symbolic or assembly, languages, which allowed programmers to specify instructions in words. High-level programming languages were also being developed at this time, such as early versions of COBOL and FORTRAN. Thanks to this rapid development new types of careers (programmer, analyst and computer systems expert) began with these second generation computers. Throughout the early 1960s, there were a number of commercially successful second generation computers used in business, universities and government from companies such as Burroughs, Control Data, Honeywell, IBM, Sperry-Rand and others. These computers also contained all the components we associate with modern computers: printers, tape storage, disk storage, memory, operating systems and stored programs described. The first computers of this generation were developed for the atomic energy industry.

Main memory (RAM) shifted from revolving magnetic drums to tiny wire-wrapped magnetic donuts called magnetic core memory. These were also the first computers that stored their instructions in their memory, which moved from a magnetic drum to magnetic core technology. This also allowed computers to become much smaller and more efficient.

The main advantage of second generation computers was the capability of storing program and the programming language.The stored program concept meant that instructions to run a computer for a specific function (known as a program) were held inside the computer's memory and could quickly be replaced by a different set of instructions for a different function. A computer could print customer invoices and minutes later design products or calculate paychecks.

Although transistors meant improvement compared to the vacuum tube, overheating was still a major drawback.The quartz rock eliminated this problem. Jack Kilby, an engineer with Texas Instruments, developed the integrated circuit (IC) in 1958.

The Third Generation/(1965-1970) Integrated Circuits — Miniaturizing the Computer

The development of the integrated circuit was the hallmark of the third generation of computers. Transistors were a tremendous breakthrough in advancing the computer. However, no one could predict that thousands even now millions of transistors (circuits) could be compacted in such a small space. The **integrated circuit** (Refer to **Fig. 1.5**) or as it is sometimes referred to as **semiconductor chip**, packs a huge number of transistors onto a single **wafer** of **silicon**. **Robert Noyce** of **Fairchild Corporation** and **Jack Kilby** of **Texas Instruments** independently discovered the amazing attributes of integrated circuits. Placing such large numbers of transistors on a single chip vastly increased the power of a single computer and lowered its cost considerably.

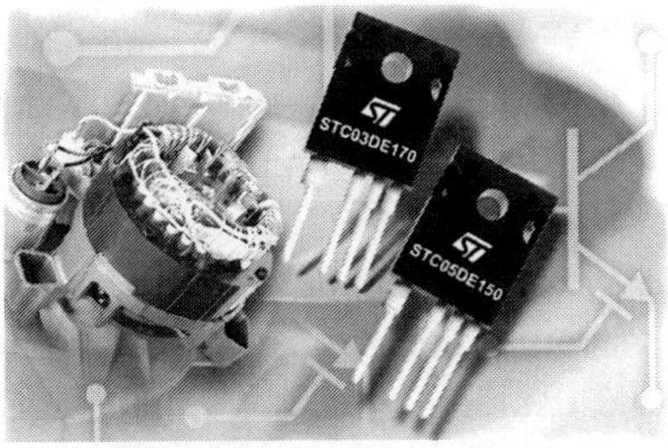

Fig. 1.5: Integrated circuits

Since the invention of integrated circuits, the number of transistors that can be placed on a single chip has **doubled** every **two** years, shrinking both the size and cost of computers even further and further enhancing its power. Most electronic devices today use some form of integrated circuits placed on printed **circuit boards** —

thin pieces of **bakelite** or **fiberglass** that have electrical connections etched onto them — sometimes called a **mother board**.

Instead of punched cards and printouts, users interacted with third generation computers through keyboards and monitors and interfaced with an operating system, which allowed the device to run many different applications at one time with a central program that monitored the memory. Computers for the first time became accessible to a mass audience because they were smaller and cheaper than their predecessors.

This was the third generation of modern computers. The IC combined three electronic components onto a small silicon disk, which was made from quartz. Scientists later managed to fit even more components on a single chip, called a **semiconductor**. As a result, computers became ever smaller as more components were squeezed onto the chip. Another third-generation development included the use of an operating system (OS) that allowed machines to run many different programs at once with a central program that monitored and coordinated the computer's memory.

Still in the sixties, 1965, precisely, the mouse was invented. However, it was not introduced to the public until the mid-eighties. Another important event was that Intel Company was founded by Robert Noyce and a few friends in 1968. They developed the first Random Access Memory (RAM) chip in 1970. It was called 1103 and had a capacity of 1 K-bit, 1024 bits.

These third generation computers could carry out instructions in billionths of a second. The size of these machines dropped to the size of small file cabinets. Yet, the single biggest advancement in the computer era was yet to be discovered.

The Fourth Generation/(1971- Present) - Microprocessors and Very Large Scale Integration (VLSI)

This generation can be characterized by both the jump to **monolithic integrated circuits** (**millions** of **transistors** put onto one integrated circuit chip, Refer to **Fig. 1.6**) and the invention of the **microprocessor** (a single chip that could do all the processing of a full-scale computer). By putting millions of transistors

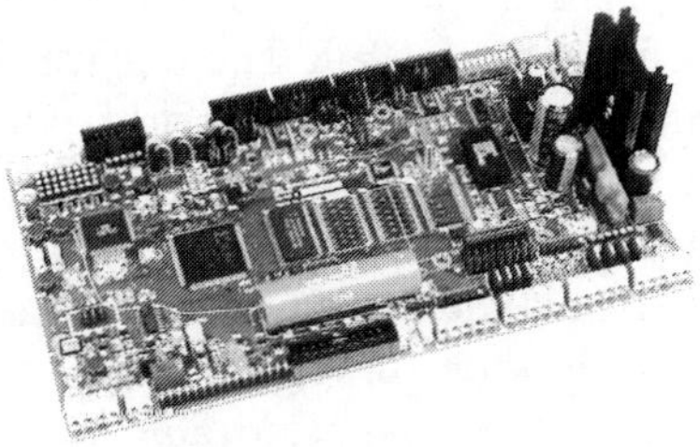

Fig. 1.6: Microprocessor

onto one single chip more calculation and faster speeds could be reached by computers. Because electricity travels about a foot in a billionth of a second, the smaller the distance the greater the speed of computers.

The microprocessor brought the fourth generation of computers, as thousands of integrated circuits were built onto a single silicon chip. What in the first generation filled an entire room could now fit in the palm of the hand. The Intel 4004 chip, developed in 1971, located all the components of the computer — from the central processing unit and memory to input/ output controls — on a single chip.

In 1981 IBM introduced its first computer for the home user and in 1984 Apple introduced the Macintosh. Microprocessors also moved out of the realm of desktop computers and into many areas of life as more and more everyday products began to use microprocessors.

As these small computers became more powerful, they could be linked together to form networks, which eventually led to the development of the Internet. Fourth generation computers also saw the development of GUIs (Graphics user interface), the mouse and hand held devices.

In the mid-seventies people started to realize how diverse the use of computers can be. They could be used not only for business but also for entertainment at home.

Pioneers in this field were Commodore, Radio Shack and Apple Computers. In the early 1980s, arcade video games such as Pac Man and home video game systems such as the Atari 2600 ignited consumer interest for more sophisticated, programmable home computers.

Soon everyday household items such as microwave ovens, television sets and automobiles with electronic fuel injection incorporated microprocessors.

This demand caused the introduction of the first Personal Computers in 1981. The biggest firm was IBM and spread the new machines all over the world. The number of personal computers in use more than doubled from 2 million in 1981 to 5.5 million in 1982. Ten years later, 65 million PCs were being used. Computers continued their trend toward a smaller size, working their way down from desktop through laptop computers (which could fit inside a briefcase) to palmtop (able to fit inside a breast pocket). IBM's biggest opponent was Apple's Macintosh, which was introduced in 1984. Its main advantage was its user-friendly application, the use of mouse instead of typing commands.

The Fifth Generation (Present and Beyond)—Artificial Intelligence (AI)

Fifth generation computing devices, based on artificial intelligence, are still in development, though there are some applications, such as voice recognition, that are being used today. The use of parallel processing and superconductors is helping to make artificial intelligence a reality. Quantum computation and molecular and nanotechnology will radically change the face of computers in years to come. The goal of fifth generation computing is to develop devices that respond to natural language input and are capable of learning and self-organization.

The development of computers has arrived at its last stage, the fifth generation. These machines are referred to as the 'computers of the future'. Two important engineering advances are parallel processing, which replaces von Neumann's single central processing unit design with a system harnessing the power of many CPUs to work as one. Another advance is superconductor technology, which allows the flow of electricity with little or no resistance, greatly improving the speed of information flow. However, this generation is in an infant state.

No one knows exactly when the improvements will stop. Companies are lauching faster and faster computers, the latest being around 3.4 GHz fast and counting. Development is so much at a high rate, that no processor can be referred to as modern for more than a month. And this fact ensures that this is one of the most profitable businesses in the world.

It is interesting or rather confusing, that it took 1200 years to develop a more modern counting device than an abacus, but our latest computers become out-of-date in just around six months. Who can keep up the pace with these improvements? And who sets the pace? Is it essential to keep it? Do we actually need a Pentium IV with 3.2 GHz, 1024 RAMs and a 100 GByte HDD? Not necessarily. But if we want to find our way in the 21st century, a computer is essential. However, the dependance on these machines could be hazardous to whole mankind. Televisions, radios, HI-FI systems, microwave ovens, walkmans, diskmans, cameras, mobile phones, digital watches, credit cards, etc. Let us imagine just one day without all the electronic gadgets.

Let's take a look at all the generations simultaneously to have an over all view (See **Table 1.1**).

IN SHORT, THE GENERAL TREND IS:

- Smaller, Faster, Lower Cost, More Reliable, More Complex
- Larger Capacity Memories, Easier Inputs and Outputs
- Easier to Use, More Flexible, Smarter, Easier Access

"...With the advent of everyday use of elaborate calculations, speed has become paramount to such a high degree that there is no machine on the market today capable of satisfying the full demand of modern computational methods. The most advanced machines have greatly reduced the time required for arriving at solutions to problems which might have required months or days by older procedures. This advance, however,, is not adequate for many problems encountered in modern scientific work and the present invention is intended to reduce to seconds such lengthy computations..."

CLASSIFICATION OF COMPUTERS

There used to be two fundamentally different types of computers:

- **Analog**
- **Digital**

Table 1.1: Generations of computers

GENERATION:	*FIRST*	*SECOND*	*THIRD*	*FOURTH*	*FIFTH*
Years:	1946-58	1959-64	1965-70	1971-?	Soon-?
Typical Machine:	UNIVAC	IBM 1400	IBM 360	Micros	Super micros?
Size:	Room	Closet	Desk	Breadbox	"Tablet"?
Circuit Device:	Vacuum tubes	Transistors	Integrated circuits	LSI[1]	VLSI[2]
Circuit Density: (#/unit)	One	100s	1,000s	Hundreds of 1,000s	Millions?
Speed: (Inst/Sec)	100s	1,000s	Millions	Tens of millions	Billions?
Reliability: (Time to fail)	Hours	Days	Weeks	Months	Years?
Main Memory Device:	Magnetic drum	Magnetic core	Magnetic Core	LSI[1] Circuits	VLSI[2], super-conductors
Memory Size:	1,000s	Tens of 1,000s	Hundreds of 1,000s	Millions	Billions?
$/Million Instructions:	$10	$1	$0.10	$0.001	$0.00001?
Input Devices:	Cards and paper tape	Cards	Key to tape/disk	Key, direct, optical	Speech touch
Output Devices:	Cards and print	Cards and print	Print and video	Print and audio/video	Graphics and voice
Software:	machine language	symbolic languages	Hi-level languages	DBMS, 4GLs SW packages	natural lang. GP packages
Some Features:	Batch process	Real-time datacomm overlaps	timeshare multiprog multiproc	Virtual memory, distributed processing	Parallel process, AI, robots

LSI[1] = Large Scale Integration of Chips with several thousand transistors. VLSI[2] = Very Large Scale Integration produced a chip containing a microprocessor — this made the development of the microcomputer possible

(Hybrid computers combine elements of both types.) In our everyday use, the term “computer” refers to digital computers, with a typical example being the common personal computer (PC). Digital computers are essentially simple machines that can understand and manipulate only series of elementary symbols: 0’s and 1’s (yes or no, true or false). The real power of a digital computer lies in the blinding speed with which it can check and manipulate these symbols, outperforming any human being. In computer lingo a bit (binary digit) is the term one uses to represent a 0 or a 1. A nibble is a series of four bits, a byte is a series of eight bits and word is used to represent multiple bytes. The trick is to arrange these series of 0’s and 1’s in such a manner that they represent whatever needs to be symbolized. For example, one could assign these 0’s and 1’s to represent a special code to instruct the machine what to do next and with what data. These designated sequences of 0’s and 1’s are called computer instructions. It is these instructions, when arranged in a structured sequence, i.e. a computer program that distinguishes the digital computer from a fast calculator. The sequence in which these instructions are executed can be altered depending on the outcome of the actions of previous instructions within the machine or input from the outside world. Instructions arrange and shuffle the bits, nibbles and bytes in such a manner that the computer can perform complex calculations and then, minutes later, help us with word processing or enable us to record variables from a monitoring device we use during anesthesia.

Computers are available in different shapes, sizes and weights, due to these different shapes and sizes they perform different sorts of jobs from one another. They differ in **size, speed of operation, amount of data that can be stored and the number of simultaneous users**.

They can also be classified in different ways. All the computers are designed by the qualified computer architectures that design these machines as their requirements.

A computer that is used in a home differs in size and shape from the computer being used in a hospital. Computers act as a server in large buildings, while the computer also differs in size and shape performing its job as a weather forecaster.

A student carrying a laptop with him to his college is different in shape and size from all the computers mentioned above.

Here we are going to introduce different classifications of computers one by one. We will discuss what are in classifications and what job they perform.

Super Computer

The biggest in size, t.he most expensive in price than any other is classified and known as super computer. It can process trillions of instructions in seconds. This computer is not used as a PC in a home neither by a student in a college.

Governments specially use this type of computer for their different calculations and heavy jobs. Different industries also use this huge computer for designing their products.

In most of the Hollywood's movies it is used for animation purposes. This kind of computer is also helpful for forecasting weather reports worldwide.

Mainframes

Another giant in computers after the super computer is mainframe, which can also process millions of instruction per second and capable of accessing billions of data. **Mainframes** allow many simultaneous users, handle typically huge databases and can perform complex mathematical operations. We find them mainly in industry, research and university computing centers.

This computer is commonly used in big hospitals, airline reservations companies and many other huge companies prefer mainframe because of its capability of retrieving data on a huge basis.

This is normally too expensive and out of reach from a salary-based person who wants a computer for his home.

This kind of computer can cost upto thousands of dollars.

Minicomputer

This computer is next in the line but offers less than mainframe in work and performance. These are the computers, which are mostly preferred by the small type of business personals, colleges, etc. **Minicomputers** can support a smaller number of simultaneous users, typically 50 to 100. These machines are primarily used by larger businesses to handle accounting, billing and inventory records.

Microcomputers

The **microcomputer** is essentially a personal or desktop computer. These desktop PCs, which dwarf the capabilities of the huge early computers, are used extensively in the home (entertainment, communication, personal databases and spreadsheets) and in all types of businesses (word processing, accounting, inventory control, research).

Personal Computers

Almost all the computer users are familiar with the personal computers. They normally know what the personal computer is and what its functions are.

This is the computer mostly preferred by the home users. These computers are lesser in cost than the computers given above and also, small in size; they are also called PCs in short for personal computers.

This computer is small in size and you can easily arrange it to fit in your single bedroom with its all accommodation. Today this is thought to be the most popular computer in all.

Notebook Computers

Having a small size and low weight the notebook is easy to carry to anywhere. A student can take it with him/her to his/her school in his/her bag with his/her book.

This is easy to carry around and preferred by students and business people to meet their assignments and other necessary tasks.

The approach of this computer is also the same as the personal computer. It can store the same amount of data and having a memory of the same size as that of a personal computer. One can say that it is the replacement of personal desktop computer.

Palmtop/Hand-held Computers

Now the computers, which can be held easily using a single hand, are available. They too have a screen generally a touch screen and are fitted with a pen like stylus for input instead of the keyboard or mouse. Handhelds are usually popular with people whose work involves the things done automatically by pointing rather than typing. These pen-based computers are known as personal data assistants (PDA). Being fitted with electronic pen like stylus, they can accept hand written input also.

Two

Operating Systems

INTRODUCTION TO THE OPERATING SYSTEM

The operating system (commonly referred to as the OS) controls the complete system and is responsible for the execution of the programs, storage of data and all other functions.

It's NEED?

The computer that consists of input devices, CPU, output devices and memory cannot produce any result if there is no interaction between the various hardware peripherals. Like any other machine, a computer also needs an operator that interacts between the hardware and the user. This job is taken care of by the Operating System.

Therefore, operating system is a system-software that makes the Central Processing Unit (CPU) co-ordinate with the other parts of the computer system to ensure smooth functioning.

Definition of an Operating system

An operating system is an integrated set of programs that is used to manage the various resources and the overall operations of the computer system.

PRIME OBJECTIVE

- Support operations of a computer system
- Improve performance and efficiency of the computer
- *Increase usability of the system making it more* **USER-FRIENDLY**
- Act as a bridge between the users and the machine.

What does an operating system do?

An operating system controls the way in which the computer system functions. In order to do this, the operating system includes programs that:

- Initialize the hardware of the computer system
- Provide basic routines for device control
- Provide for the management, scheduling and interaction of tasks
- Maintain system integrity and handle errors.

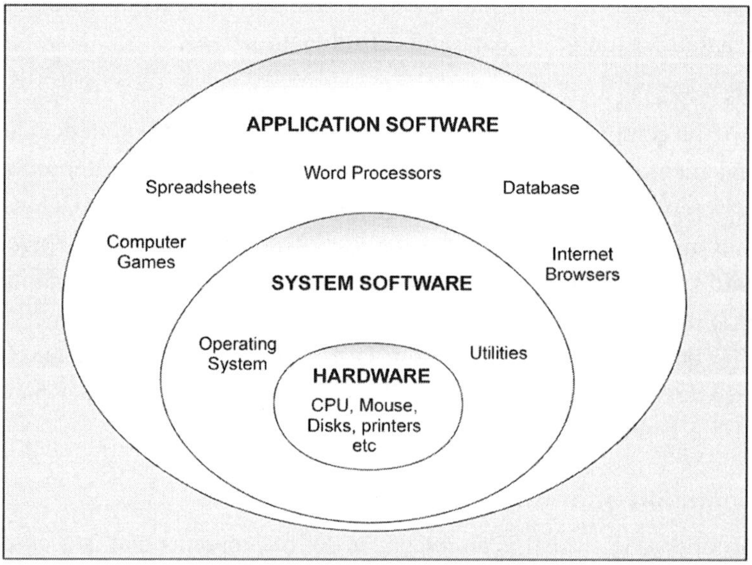

Fig 2.1: Computer schema

Where are operating systems found?

There are many types of operating systems, the complexity of which varies depending upon what type of functions are provided and what the system is being used for. Some systems are responsible for managing many users on a network. Other operating systems (Refer to **Fig. 2.1**) do not manage user programs at all. These are typically found in hardware devices like petrol pumps, airplanes, video recorders, washing machines and car engines.

FUNCTIONS AND SERVICES

Operating System Utilities

The operating system consists of hundreds of thousands of lines of program code and is stored on the hard disk. Portions of the operating system are loaded into computer system memory (RAM) when needed. Utilities are provided for:

- Managing files and documents
- Development of programs and software
- Communicating between people and with other computer systems
- Managing user requirements for programs, storage space and priority.

Operating System Interfaces

In addition, the operating system provides each user with an interface that accepts, interprets and executes user commands or programs. This interface is commonly called a SHELL or command line interpreter (CLI). In some systems this might be a simple text mode line-by-line entry using keywords (such as MS-DOS or UNIX), in other systems it might be highly graphical using windows and a pointing device such as a mouse (such as Windows XP).

COMPONENTS OF AN OPERATING SYSTEM

What are the various parts of an operating system?

In this section we look at that part of the operating system that is responsible for running programs, called the real-time executive or kernel.

An operating system for a large-scale computer that is used by many people at once is a very complex system. It contains many millions of lines of instructions (commands that the computer executes) written by programmers. To make operating systems easier to write, they are constructed as a series of modules (programs), each module responsible for one function. Typical modules in a larger multi-user operating system could be:

- Kernel (also known as the executive)
- Process manager
- Scheduler
- File manager.

What is a real-time executive?

The core of all operating systems is called a REAL-TIME EXECUTIVE (also known as the kernel). Some of the functions that it performs are:

- Switching between programs
- Hardware device control and programming
- Memory management
- Process management
- Scheduling (deciding what programs to run)
- Inter-process communication
- Processing of exceptions and interrupts.

Our simple 'security monitoring system' would not have all of the above, as it would probably be a single task system, running only one program. As such, it would not need to perform scheduling of more than one program or allow communication to take place between programs (called inter-process communication). Memory management would be unnecessary, as the program would easily fit into the available memory of the computer.

An operating system designed to handle a large number of people would need a real-time executive that performs all of the above. User programs are generally stored on disk, thus need to be loaded into memory before being executed. This presents the need for memory management, as the memory of the computer would need to be searched for a free area in which to load a persons program into. When the user is finished running the program, the memory consumed by it would need to be freed up and made available for another user when required.

Process scheduling and management is also necessary, so that all programs would be executed and run fairly. There is no point if a program by a specific user runs to such an extent that it denies the running of any other programs, making every other user wait. In addition, some programs might need to be executed more frequently than others, for example, checking network communications or printing. Some programs may need to be temporarily halted, then restarted again later, so this introduces the need for inter-program communication.

TYPES AND CLASSIFICATION: SINGLE USER, MULTIPLE USERS

What is a single-user operating system?

We are all familiar with the concept of sitting down at a computer system and writing documents or performing some task such as writing a letter. In this instance there is one keyboard and one monitor that you interact with.

Operating systems such as Windows 95, Windows NT Workstation and Windows 2000 professional are essentially single-user operating systems. They provide you the capability to perform tasks on the computer system such as writing programs and documents, printing and accessing files.

Consider a typical home computer. There is a single keyboard and mouse that accept input commands and a single monitor to display information output. There may also be a printer for the printing of documents and images.

In essence, a single-user operating system provides access to the computer system by a single user at a time. If another user needs access to the computer system, they must wait till the current user finishes what they are doing and leaves.

Students in computer labs at colleges or universities often experience this. You might also have experienced this at home, where you want to use the computer but someone else is currently using it. You have to wait for them to finish before you can use the computer system.

What is a multi-user operating system?

A multi-user operating system lets more than one user access the computer system at one time. Access to the computer system is normally provided via a network, so that users access the computer remotely using a terminal or other computer (**Fig. 2.2**).

Today, these terminals are generally personal computers and use a network to send and receive information to the multi-user computer system. Examples of multi-user operating systems are UNIX, Linux (a UNIX clone) and mainframes such as the IBM AS400.

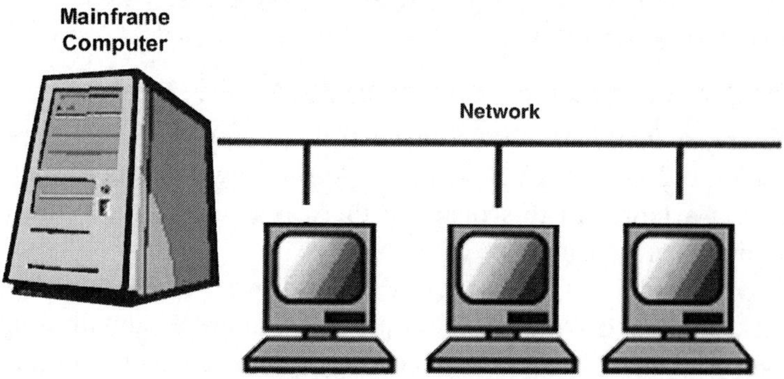

Fig. 2.2: Multi-user architecture

The operating system for a large multi-user computer system with many terminals is much more complex than a single-user operating system. It must manage and run all user requests, ensuring they do not interfere with each other. Devices that are serial in nature (devices which can only be used by one user at a time, like printers and disks) must be shared amongst all those requesting them (so that all the output documents are not jumbled up). If each user tried to send their document to the printer at the same time, the end result would be garbage. Instead, documents are sent to a queue and each document is printed in its entirety before the next document to be printed is retrieved from the queue. When you wait inline at the cafeteria to be served you are in a queue. Imagine that all the people in the queue are documents waiting to be printed and the cashier at the end of the queue is the printer.

Advantages and Problems with Multi-user Operating Systems

The advantage of having a multi-user operating system is that normally the hardware is very expensive and it lets a number of users share this expensive resource. This means the cost is divided amongst the users. It also makes better use of the resources. Since the resources are shared, they are more likely to be in use than sitting idle being unproductive.

One problem with multi-user computer systems is that as more users access it, the performance becomes slower and slower. Another disadvantage is the cost of hardware, as a multi-user operating system requires a lot of disk space and memory. In addition, the actual software for multi-user operating systems tend to cost more than single-user operating systems.

What is a multi-tasking operating system?

A multi-tasking operating system provides the ability to run more than one program at once. For example, a user could be running a word processing package, printing a document, copying files to the floppy disk and backing up selected files to a tape unit. Each of these tasks the user is doing appears to be running at the same time.

A multi-tasking operating system has the advantage of letting the user run more than one task at once, so this leads to increased productivity. The disadvantage is that more programs that are run by the user, the more memory that is required.

What are the different types of operating systems?

Operating systems are divided into categories that define their characteristics. Modern systems may use combinations of those described below (**Table 2.1**).

Some characteristics of an operating system are:

- Whether multiple programs can run on it simultaneously: *multi-tasking*
- Whether it can take advantage of multiple processors: *multi-processing*

Table 2.1: Types of operating systems

BATCH	The earliest type, allowed only one program to run at a time. The program was entered into the computer, then run till completed. The data used by the program could not be modified whilst the program was running. Any errors in the program or data mean starting all over again.
INTERACTIVE	These allow the modification and entry of data whilst the program is running. Typical systems are airline reservations and languages such as BASIC.
TIME-SHARING **MULTI-USER**	These share the computer system amongst more than one user and employ pre-emptive scheduling techniques.
MULTI-TASKING	More than one process may be executed at once. The processor is switched rapidly between the processes. A user may run more than one process at a time.
REAL-TIME	Primarily used in process control, telecommunications, etc. The OS monitors various inputs which affect the execution of processes, changing the computers model of the environment, thus affecting the outputs, within a guaranteed time period (usually less than 1 second).
MULTI-PROCESSOR	A computer that has more than one processor dedicated to running processes.
EMBEDDED	An embedded operating system means the operating system is self-contained in the device and resident in ROM. Typical systems that use embedded operating systems are household appliances, car management systems, traffic control systems and energy management systems.

- Whether multiple users can run programs on it simultaneously: *multi-user*
- Whether it can reliably prevent application programs from directly accessing hardware devices: *protected*
- Whether it has built-in support for graphics.
- Whether it has built-in support for networks.

Some popular operating systems are:

- **UNIX:** multi-tasking, multi-processing, multi-user, protected, with built-in support for networking but not graphics.
- **Windows NT:** multi-tasking, multi-processing, single-user, protected, with built-in support for networking and graphics.
- **Windows 95/98/XP:** multi-tasking, multi-processing, single-user, unprotected, with built-in support for networking and graphics.
- **Windows 3.x:** single-tasking, single-processing, single-user, unprotected, with built-in support for graphics but not networking.
- **DOS:** single-tasking, single-processing, single-user, unprotected with no built-in support for graphics or networking.
- **NetWare:** multi-tasking, multi-processing, single-user, unprotected, with built-in support for networking but not graphics.

MOST POPULAR OS: MS-DOS AND WINDOWS

Introduction to DOS

DOS, short for *Disk Operating System*, is a program which acts as an interface between the user and the computer hardware. DOS allows manipulation of files and programs by interpreting and processing the commands typed by the user. The DOS software is automatically copied from secondary storage (a floppy disk or the hard drive) into the microcomputer's memory whenever the computer is turned on or booted. DOS is not an application package that you start and then exit when done. The operating system runs from the moment you turn the microcomputer on until you turn the machine off. The advantage and disadvantages of DOS are listed in **Table 2.2**.

Table 2.2: DOS-Pros and Cons

Pros	***Cons***
Dedicates almost all memory to applications	No multi-tasking capabilities
Speedy boots	Fewdll's means larger installations
Shells are widespread and popular	The older versions of windows are being replaced with newer versions
Simple interface	Few programs are now supported

Basic DOS Structure

There are actually several levels to DOS. At the lowest level is the **BIOS** (Basic Input/Output System) which is responsible for managing devices like the keyboards and disk drives at the simplest possible level (e.g. the BIOS lets you say things like "get me sector 5 of track 3 from disk drive 1"). This is done partly by software in ROM (read-only memory) and partly by BIOS extensions which are loaded when the system first starts up (with MS-DOS, these are in a file called IO.SYS; on PC-DOS they are in IBMBIO.COM).

The second layer provides a set of higher level services implemented using the low-level BIOS services; you can now refer to disk drive 1 as "drive A:" and instead of referring to specific sectors or tracks you can refer to files by name (e.g. LETTER.TXT). You can also treat devices as if they were named files, so that for example you can use the name PRN: to refer to the printer. In other words, this level provides a **file system** (you can refer to files by name and let DOS worry about translating the name into a physical location) as well as some device independence (you do not have to differentiate storing text in a file from sending it to the printer). This layer of the system is implemented by another file which is loaded when the system first starts up (the file is called MSDOS.SYS on MS-DOS systems and IBMDOS.COM on PC-DOS systems).

The third layer is the **command interpreter** (or **shell**), which is what most people think of as DOS (it's not, but it's what you interact with when you use the computer, so it's an understandable confusion). This is contained in another file called COMMAND.COM, which is just an ordinary program that is started. The shell's job is to display a **command prompt** on the screen to let you know you're supposed to type something, then to read a line of text that you type and to interpret it as a command, which usually involves loading another program into memory and running it. When it's finished doing this, it displays another prompt and waits for you to type in another command.

The File System

Before we go any further, it would be a good idea to look at the DOS file system. The **file system** lets us store information in named **files**. You can call a file anything you like which might help you remember what it contains as long as you follow certain basic rules:

1. File names can be upto 8 characters long. You can use letters and digits but only a few punctuation marks (! $ % # ~ @ - ( ) _ { }). You cannot exceed 8 characters or use spaces or characters like * or ? or +. Names are case-insensitive, i.e. it does not matter whether you use capitals or lowercase letters; "A" and "a" are treated as the same thing.
2. File names can also have an **extension** of upto three characters which describes the type of file. There are some standard extensions, but you don't have to use them. Examples include COM and EXE for executable programs, TXT for text files, BAK for backup copies of files or CPP for C^{++} program files. The extension is separated by a dot from the rest of the filename.

For example, a file called FILENAME.EXT has an 8-character name (FILENAME) followed by a three-character extension (.EXT). You could also refer to it as filename.txt since case does not matter, but I'm going to use names in capitals for emphasis throughout this document.

Files are stored in **directories**; a directory is actually just a special type of file which holds a list of the files within it. Since a directory is a file, you can have directories within directories. Directory names also follow the same naming rules as other files, but although they can have an extension they are not normally given one (just an 8-character name).

The system keeps track of your **current directory** and if you just refer to a file using a name like FILENAME.EXT it's assumed you mean a file of that name in the current directory. You can specify a **pathname** to identify a file which includes the directory name as well; the directory is separated from the rest of the name by a backslash ("\"). For example, a file called LETTER1.TXT in a directory called LETTERS can be referred to as LETTERS\LETTER1.TXT (assuming that the current directory contains the LETTERS directory as a subdirectory). If LETTERS contains a subdirectory called PERSONAL, which in turn contains a file called ARJUN.TXT, you would refer to this file as LETTERS\PERSONAL\ARJUN.TXT (i.e. look in the LETTERS directory for PERSONAL\ARJUN.TXT, which in turn involves looking in the PERSONAL subdirectory for the file ARJUN.TXT).

Every disk has a **root directory** which is the main directory that everything else is part of. The root directory is called "\", so you can use **absolute pathnames** which don't depend on what your current directory is. A name like \LETTERS\LETTER1.TXT always refers to the same file regardless of which directory you happen to be working in at the time; the "\" at the beginning means "start looking in th.e root directory", so \LETTERS\LETTER1.TXT means "look in the root directory of the disk for a subdirectory called LETTERS, then look in this subdirectory for a file called LETTER1.TXT". Leaving out the "\" at the beginning makes this a **relative pathname** whose meaning is relative to the current directory at the time.

If you want to refer to a file on another disk, you can put a letter identifying the disk at the beginning of the name separated from the rest of the name by a colon (":"). For example, A:\LETTER1.TXT refers to a file called LETTER1.TXT in the root directory of drive A. DOS keeps track of the current directory on each disk separately, so a relative pathname like A:\LETTER1.TXT refers to a file called LETTER1.TXT in the currently-selected directory on drive A.

For convenience, all directories (except root directories) contain two special names: "." refers to the directory itself and ".." refers to the parent directory (i.e. the directory that contains this one). For example, if the current directory is \LETTERS\PERSONAL, the name ".." refers to the directory \LETTERS, "..\BUSINESS" refers to \LETTERS\BUSINESS and "..\.." refers to the root directory "\".

The AUTOEXEC.BAT File

The file C:\AUTOEXEC.BAT is a special one, because when the system is first started the command interpreter will automatically execute this file as a batch file (hence the name). This is where to put all your system startup commands; for example, setting the path, loading your keyboard and mouse driver, running a virus checker or whatever. Whenever you install any new DOS software, you'll need to check whether you need to update this file (and if you do, you'll either need to restart the system or type C:\AUTOEXEC.BAT to re-execute it before any of the changes will take effect). You'll often need to update your path to include the directory where your new software was installed. Some software will do this automatically and amazingly often it will get it wrong or do it in such a way that something else no longer works.

Basic Commands

Each DOS command described in the following section uses standard command description notation.

Notation	Interpretation
UPPER CASE	keywords (do not have to typed in upper case) lower case values supplied by the user.
[ ]	optional values; the square brackets are not part of the command.
{ }	one of the enclosed elements must be chosen; the brace (brackets are not part of the command).
ITEM1|ITEM2	choose one of the elements in the list and type it as part of the command.
Drive:	drive specification to be supplied by the user. Must be specified if you are using a file that is not on the current drive.

Path	a sequence of directory names to be supplied by the user.
Filename	name of file with the filename extension.

CHDIR or CD

Change the current directory to the specified drive and path.
Format:

CHDIR path

CD path

where: path *is one of:*

- a directory path
- \ (the root directory)
- .. (the parent directory)

Examples:

cd\

Change to the root directory.

cd ..

Change to the parent of the current directory.

cd\wp

Change to the WP directory one level below the root.

cd programs

Change to the PROGRAMS directory if you are currently in the parent directory PROJECTS; if you are in any other directory you will get an error.

CHKDSK

Analyzes the directories, files and file allocation table on the disk in the specified drive and produces a disk and primary memory status report on the screen. If CHKDSK is run with the fix option, repairs may cause a loss of information. Consequently, DOS will ask if you want the 'lost chains' converted into files. If you answer yes, each lost chain is converted to a file named *file###.chk*. These files can be checked for lost data that you need. If you answer no, the contents of the lost chains are not saved to files.
Format:

*CHKDSK [*drive:*][*pathname*] [/F]*

where/F fixes errors on the disk

Example:

chkdsk a:

Check the status of the disk in the A: drive.

CLS

Clear the display screen, leaving the DOS prompt at the upper left corner of the screen.

Format:

CLS

COPY

Copy one or more files to another location. The source file is not erased. If the destination file already exists, the old contents are overwritten. Can be used to concatenate (join together) files. Copy can be used to copy files to devices such as the printer (PRN) or the console (CON). The console is an old-fashioned term and actually refers to your screen. On the network, you must select a printer with PRINTER before copying to PRN. The printer selected and the file format must match!

Format:

COPY [*drive*:][*path*] *source filename* [*drive*:][*path*] [*destination filename*] [/V]

COPY [*drive*:][*path*] *source filename* PRN

COPY [*drive*:][*path*] *source filename* CON

where: /V verifies the sectors written on the disk are recorded properly.

Examples:

copy oldfile.doc newfile.doc/v

Create a new file called NEWFILE.DOC, which is the same as OLDFILE.DOC. Both files are in the current directory.

copy c:\wp\data\manual.doc c:\projects\data\manual.doc

Copy MANUAL.DOC in the \WP\DATA directory to the \PROJECTS\DATA directory.

copy a:*.*
Copy all files in the current directory of A: to the current drive and directory. The current directory cannot be the root directory on A:. A file cannot be copied onto itself.
copy test1.dat con
Copy TEST1.DAT to the screen if \PROJECTS\DATA is the current directory.
copy test1.dat+test2.dat fulltest.dat
Concatenate the contents of TEST1.DAT and TEST2.DAT and place the result into FULLTEST.DAT in the current directory (\PROJECTS\DATA for this example).

DATE

Display current date and prompt for new date. Pressing <ENTER> at the prompt leaves date unchanged (used to check current date).

Format:

DATE [mm-dd-yy]
where:

- mm = month (1-12)
- dd = day (1-31)
- yy = year (00-99) or (2000-2099)

DEL or ERASE

Delete files from disk. Subdirectories cannot be deleted with DEL or ERASE, use RMDIR (ReMove DIRrectory).

Format:

DEL [*drive*:][*path*]*filename* [/P]
ERASE [*drive*:][*path*]*filename* [/P]
where: /P prompts you before a deletion actually occurs with a *filename, Delete (Y/N)?* message.

NOTE: Caution! Take care when using wildcards (described ahead in this chapter). Valuable files may be lost through poor choice of wildcards.

Examples:

del file.ext

Delete FILE.EXT from the current directory.

del *.*

Delete all files in current directory. Due to the possible danger, the system will ask you whether you are sure. Reply appropriately.

del c:\wp\data*.bk1

Delete all files with the .BK1 extension in the \WP\DATA directory on the C: drive.

del test?.dat

Delete all files in the current directory with a filename length of 5 characters of which the first 4 characters are TEST and which have the .DAT extension.

DIR

List directory contents. Files are listed with their size in bytes and their last modification date.

Format:

DIR [*drive*:][*path*][*filename*] [/P] [/W]

where:

- /P pauses after each screen is filled (23 lines)
- /W wide listing; lists only filenames in four columns across the screen.

Examples:

dir

List all files in current directory. (same as DIR *.*)

dir *.doc

List all files in current directory with the .DOC extension.

dir c:\wp*.* /p

List all files in the \WP subdirectory on the C: drive and pauses at the end of each screen.

DISKCOPY

Copy an entire floppy disk and format the target floppy disk if necessary. Use only to copy to similar disks of the same density, i.e. 5.25 inch low density to 5.25 inch low density or 3.5 inch high density to 3.5 inch high density, not 5.25 inch to 3.5 inch.

Format:

DISKCOPY [*source drive*: [*target drive*:]]

Examples:

diskcopy a: b:

Format the disk in drive B: if required, then copy the contents of the disk in drive A: to the disk in drive B:, assuming that they are compatible in size and density.

diskcopy

Uses the default drive as both source and target and prompts you to change disks as required. The current default drive must be a floppy drive.

diskcopy a: a:

Used to copy disks if you only have one floppy drive. DOS will prompt you for the source disk and then the target disk.

FORMAT

Prepare a new disk for use by organizing the tracks and sectors on the disk, creating space for a file directory and locking out defective disk areas. All floppy disks must be formatted before information can be stored on them. New disks are typically unformatted.

Format:

FORMAT *drive*: [/S]

FORMAT A: /N:9 /T:80 [/S] *** see explanation in first example

where:

- /S will copy system files to new disk
- /T:# number of tracks on the disk
- /N:# number of sectors per track

NOTE: Caution! Formatting a disk will destroy any files already on it, so use this command with caution. If your default drive is a hard drive, typing in FORMAT with no drive designator will cause DOS to reformat the hard drive. The machine will not be useable. You do not want to do this by accident!

Examples:

format a: /s

Format a floppy disk in the A: drive and copy the operating system files to the disk. You will be able to boot-up from this floppy.

format a: /n:9 /t:80

Format a double density 3.5" disk to 9 sectors and 80 tracks. On the network, the floppy drive defaults to high density (18 sectors and 80 tracks). This command gives DOS the information to format in double density rather than high density.

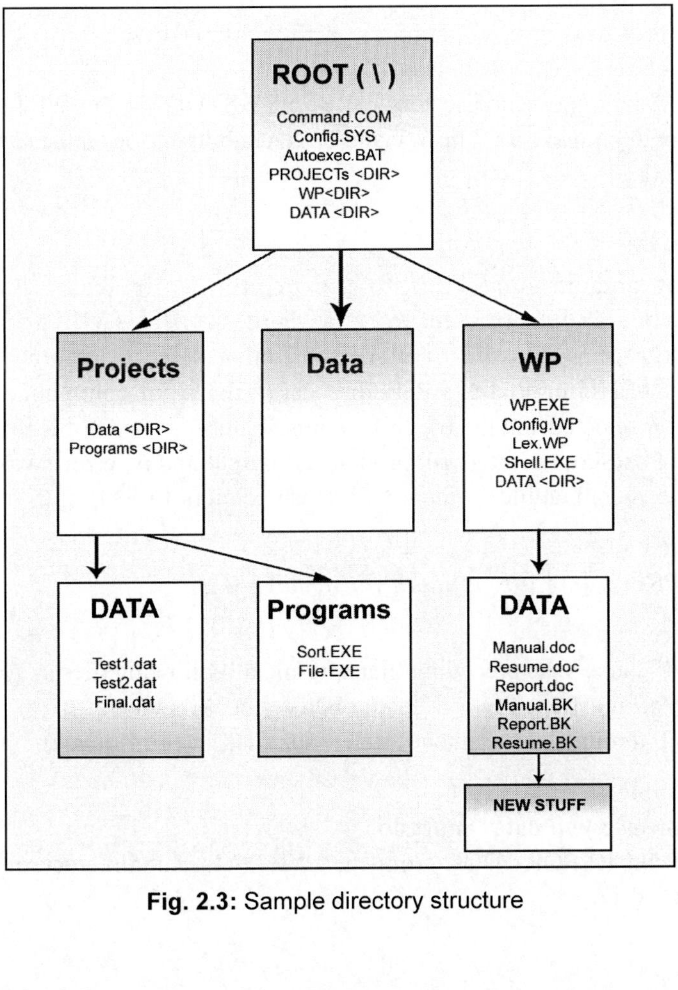

Fig. 2.3: Sample directory structure

If you have a high density floppy disk use FORMAT a:

MKDIR or MD

Make a new subdirectory with the specified pathname (Refer to **Fig. 2.3**).

Format:

MKDIR [*drive*:]*path*

MD [*drive*:]*path*

Examples:

mkdir data

Make a new subdirectory called DATA in the current directory (root directory in example) on the current drive.

mkdir c:\wp\data\newstuff.

Make a new subdirectory called NEWSTUFF in the WP\DATA path on drive C:. The WP and DATA subdirectories must already exist.

PRINT

Print one or more files to the printer while leaving your microcomputer free to work with other files (will print in background). On the network, you must select a printer with PRNMENU or PRINTER before using the print command. The printer selected and the file format must match! An ASCII file printed on a PostScript printer will produce no output and no error message. Some incompatible formats will cause printers to lock up!

Format:

PRINT [/T] [*drive*:][*path*][*filename*] [/C]

where:

- /C cancels the preceding filename and all following files in queue. You must specify a filename before the /C switch.
- /T terminates the queue (delete all files in print queue).

Example:

print c:\wp\data\report.doc

Print REPORT.DOC from the \WP\DATA subdirectory on the C: drive.

RENAME or REN

Change the name of a file(s).

Format:

RENAME [*drive*:][*path*]*oldfilename newfilename*
REN [*drive*:][*path*]*oldfilename newfilename*

Examples:

rename c:\wp\data\report.doc final.doc
Rename the file REPORT.DOC, in the \WP\DATA directory, to FINAL.DOC.
rename manual.doc oldman.doc
Rename the file MANUAL.DOC, in the current directory, to OLDMAN.DOC. This command will only work if the current directory is C:\WP\DATA; otherwise, you will get a file not found error.

RMDIR or RD

Remove a directory. The directory can only be removed if it contains no files or lower level subdirectories. Remove files using the DEL or ERASE command.

Format:

RMDIR [*drive*:]*path*
RD [*drive*:]*path*

Examples:

rmdir \data
Remove the DATA directory, if it is empty.
rmdir c:\wp\data\newstuff
Remove the NEWSTUFF subdirectory, if it is empty.

TIME

Display current time and prompts for new time. Pressing <ENTER> at the prompt leaves time unchanged (used to see current time).

Format:

TIME [hh:mm[:ss[.xx]]]

where:

- hh = hours (0-23)
- mm = minutes (0-59)
- ss = seconds (0-59)
- xx = hundredths of seconds (0-99)

  If ss and xx are omitted, they default to zero.

TYPE

Display a file on the screen (by default) or redirect the file to another file or to the printer (PRN).

Format:

TYPE [*drive*:][*path*]*filename*
TYPE [*drive*:][*path*]*filename* > PRN
TYPE [*drive*:][*path*]*filename* > *filename2*

Example:

type autoexec.bat

Display the contents of the file *AUTOEXEC.BAT* in the current directory (root directory in example) on the screen.

XCOPY

Copy files including, if desired, files from child subdirectories. XCOPY reads as many sour.

Wildcards

In some situations it's useful to be able to specify sets of files to be operated on by a single command. For example, you might want to delete all files with the extension ".TXT". You can do this like so:

DEL *.TXT

The star "*" matches any name at all. You can read it as "anything .TXT", although if I had to read this command out loud I'd probably say "del star-dot-text". Anyway, what it means is that any file whose name matches the pattern *.TXT (any file with a .TXT extension) will be deleted. You can do more sophisticated things:

COPY NOTE*.TXT NOTES

will copy any file whose name begins with NOTE (i.e. NOTE followed by anything) and has a .TXT extension to the NOTES subdirectory. The star is referred to as a wildcard by analogy with the role of a Joker in some card games, where the Joker can be used as any other card. The command

DEL *.*

will delete all the files in the current directory (all files with any name and any extension). Since this is obviously risky, you'll be prompted with a message that says "Are you sure (Y/N)?". If you are sure, type Y for "yes"; if not type N for "no". A non-obvious use of this technique is allowed by the REN (rename) command:

REN *.TXT *.LST

will rename all files with a .TXT extension to files with the same name but a .LST extension instead. A limitation of this technique is that you can only use a star as a wildcard at the end of the name or extension part of a filename; you might think that you could delete all files whose name ends with X like this:

DEL *X.*

Unfortunately this has the same effect as

DEL *.*

since the star matches everything upto the end of the name and the X after that is just ignored. You can use a question mark to match a single character:

DEL ?X.*

This will match any file whose name consists of any single character followed by an X with any extension. To delete any files whose name ends with X would actually require a whole sequence of commands:

DEL X.*
DEL ?X.*
DEL ??X.*
DEL ???X.*
DEL ????X.*
DEL ?????X.*
DEL ??????X.*
DEL ???????X.*

This deletes all files whose name is X, then all files whose name is any one character followed by X, then all files whose name is any two characters followed by X and so on upto any seven characters followed by X.

Three

Introduction to Database

INTRODUCTION

All of us are familiar with the term ***data***. In fact, unknowingly we come across data in our day-to-day life everyday. The age of a person, price of potatoes, number of students in a school, pin code of a city, etc. are some examples of data. In our lives we have to remember a lot of data. Remembering information on a few things is easy. But when the amount of information grows out of the human brain's retention ability, we can no longer remember or reproduce information efficiently. For example, you may be in a position to tell the age, height, complexion, income, educational qualification, residential address, etc. of your close friends. But it is very difficult for you to memorize such detailed information for a large number of individuals. Let us consider the example of AIIMS, New Delhi. Every year, thousands of patients get admitted to the hospital. But if you are asked to memorize the dates of birth, medical history and medication details of all these patients, it will not be possible for you!

To deal with such problems we construct a database. We arrange all information about the subject (patients in this case) in a tabular form. We keep all the records so that if I am asked, "How many patients are there in the ICU?" I am in a position to answer.

WHAT IS A DATABASE?

Let us begin with the concept 'database' and its management. Database is a collection of information in a structured way. We can say that it is a collection of a group of facts. Your personal address book is a database of names you like to keep track of, such as personal friends and members of your family.

Table 3.1: Student Information

ROLL NO	*NAME*	*DOB*	*SEX*	*ADDRESS*	*SUBJECTS*
9721001	Abhimanyu	31.12.1985	M	C36, Sector 2, Mhow	Mechanical
9721002	Sharon Singh	16.05.1984	M	At/Po. Delhi	Electronics and Telecommunication
9732012	Vikram Duggal	03.01.1986	M	A31, Gurgaon	Information Technology
9724004	Pulkit Saxena	23.11.1985	M	12A, Sheikh Sarai-I, Jaipur	Mechanical
9715023	Yolando Pereira	07.09.1985	M	96, Malviya Nagar, Goa	Computers

Let us look into an example of information on students in a class. A sample of 5 students is presented in Table 3.1. We have given 6 items of information on every student, namely, Roll No, Name, Date of birth, Sex, Postal address and Subjects offered by the student.

The table contains required details about each student. There are six pieces of information on each student. They are Roll No, Name, Date of birth, Sex, Address and Subjects. Each piece of information in database is called a ***Field***. We can define ***field* as *the smallest unit in a database***. Each field represents one and only one characteristic of an event or item. Thus there are six fields in this database.

If you take a close look at all these fields, they are not of the same type. Date of birth is *date* type whereas Name is *character* type. In database there can be five categories of fields. They are:

- **Numeric**
- **Character**
- **Logic**
- **Memo**
- **Date**

We will discuss about each type of field in detail later on in this lesson. First let us be familiar with another concept that we will use frequently. All the related fields for a particular event is called a ***Record*** (Refer to **Fig. 3.1**). In the example above, all six fields taken together for a particular student is called a record of that student. Hence, since there are six students there are six records. Thus, **we can define record as *a collection of logically related fields.***

Now we are in a position to define database in a formal manner. We can say that ***a database is a collection of logically related records***. In other words a database is a collection of database files

9715023	Yolando Pereira	07.09.1980	M	96, Malviya Nagar, Goa	Computers

Fig. 3.1: Example of a record

and each database file is a collection of records.

The task before us is creation of a database and its management. *Data management* involves creating, modifying, deleting and adding data in files and using this data to generate reports or answer queries. The software that allows us to perform these functions easily is called a *Data Base Management System* (DBMS). Using a DBMS files can be retrieved easily and effectively.

FIELD TYPES AND WIDTHS

In the beginning I had mentioned that there are five types of fields. Let us discuss them in detail now.

1. **Character:** This type of field contains textual matter. For example, name, address, special symbols, numbers and blank spaces. Character field can contain upto 256 characters or bytes. In Figure 3.1 the fields *Name*, *Address*, *Sex* and *Subjects* are character types.
2. **Numeric:** This type of field contains integers or decimal numbers, either positive or negative. The maximum length of numeric field is upto 19 digits long.
3. **Date:** Date fields are 8 characters long. It is in the form of MM/DD/YY where MM is the month, DD is the day of the month and YY is the year. In Figure 3.1 the field *Date of Birth* is of date type.
4. **Logical/Boolean:** It contains either a 'true' or 'false' (YES or NO) value. Its length is one character or one byte.

5. **Memo:** Memo fields are used to store large block of text or tabular information. The field width of memo field is up to 5000 characters or bytes.

DATA, INFORMATION AND ITS PROCESSING?

Data is a collection of facts, which are unorganized. Once the data has been processed and organized into something meaningful. It is called **Information**.

Data Processing is defined as a series of actions or operations that convert data into useful information. The data processing system is used to include the resourced such as people, procedures and devices that are used to accomplish the processing of data for producing desirable output. Data is the raw material for information and just as raw materials are transformed into finished products by a manufacturing process, Database Management System (DBMS) transforms this data into meaningful information.

DATABASE MANAGEMENT SYSTEMS

1. A **database management system** (DBMS) or simply a **database system** (DBS), consists of:
   - A collection of interrelated and persistent data (usually referred to as the **database** (DB)).
   - A set of application programs used to access, update and manage that data (which form the data management system (MS)).
2. The goal of a DBMS is to provide an environment that is both **convenient** and **efficient** to use in:
   - Retrieving information from the database.
   - Storing information into the database.
3. Databases are usually designed to manage **large** bodies of information. This involves
   - Definition of structures for information storage (data modeling).
   - Provision of mechanisms for the manipulation of information (file and systems structure, query processing).
   - Providing for the safety of information in the database (crash recovery and security).
   - Concurrency control if the system is shared by users.

PURPOSE OF DATABASE SYSTEMS

1. To see why database management systems are necessary, let's look at a typical "file-processing system" supported by a conventional operating system.
   The application is a savings bank:
   - Savings account and customer records are kept in permanent system files.
   - Application programs are written to manipulate files to perform the following tasks:
     - Debit or credit an account.
     - Add a new account.
     - Find an account balance.
     - Generate monthly statements.
2. Development of the system proceeds as follows:
   - New application programs must be written as the need arises.
   - New permanent files are created as required.
   - **But** over a long period of time files may be in different formats and
   - Application programs may be in different languages.
3. So we can see there are problems with the straight file-processing approach:
   - **Data redundancy and inconsistency**
     - Same information may be duplicated in several places.
     - All copies may not be updated properly.
   - **Difficulty in accessing data**
     - May have to write a new application program to satisfy an unusual request.
     - For example, find all customers with the same postal code.
     - Could generate this data manually, but it is a long job.
   - **Data isolation**
     - Data in different files.
     - Data in different formats.
     - Difficult to write new application programs.
   - **Multiple users**
     - Want concurrency for faster response time.
     - Need protection for concurrent updates.

    - For example, two customers withdrawing funds from the same account at the same time — account has $500 in it and they withdraw $100 and $50. The result could be $350, $400 or $450 if no protection is provided.
- **Security problems**
    - Every user of the system should be able to access only the data they are permitted to see.
    - For example, payroll people only handle employee records and cannot see customer accounts; tellers only access account data and cannot see payroll data.
    - Difficult to enforce this with application programs.
- **Integrity problems**
    - Data may be required to satisfy constraints.
    - For example, no account balance below $25.00.
    - Again, difficult to enforce or to change constraints with the file-processing approach.

These problems and others led to the development of **database management systems**.

DATA ABSTRACTION

1. The major purpose of a database system is to provide users with an **abstract view** of the system. The system hides certain details of how data is stored and created and maintained. Complexity should be hidden from database users.
2. There are several levels of abstraction:

Physical Level

- How the data are stored.
- For example, index, B-tree, hashing.
- Lowest level of abstraction.
- Complex low-level structures described in detail.

Conceptual Level

- Next, higher, level of abstraction.
- *Describes* what *data are stored.*
- Describes the relationships among data.
- Database administrator level.

View Level

- Highest level.
- *Describes* part *of the database for a particular group of users.*
- Can be many different views of a database.
- For example, tellers in a bank get a view of customer accounts, but not of payroll data.

  Figure 3.2 illustrates the three levels.

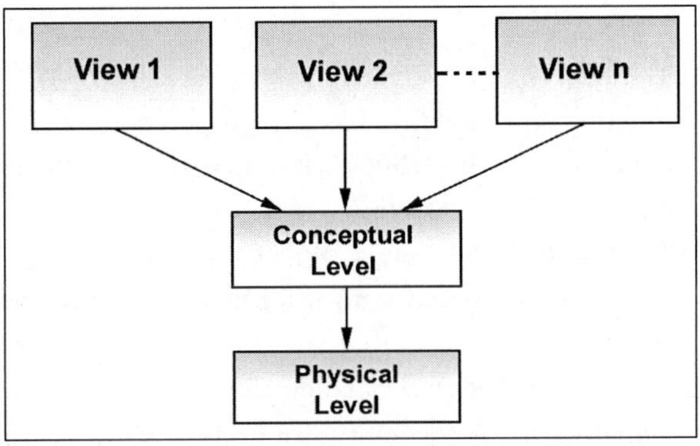

Fig. 3.2: The three levels of data abstraction

DATA MODELS

Data models are a collection of conceptual tools for describing data, data relationships, data semantics and data constraints. There are three different groups:

1. Object-based Logical Models.
2. Record-based Logical Models.
3. Physical Data Models.

OBJECT-BASED LOGICAL MODELS

Object-based logical models:

- Describe data at the conceptual and view levels.
- Provide fairly flexible structuring capabilities.
- Allow one to specify data constraints explicitly.
- Over 30 such models, including
    - Entity-relationship model.
    - Object-oriented model.
    - Binary model.
    - Semantic data model.
    - Infological model.
    - Functional data model.

At this point, we'll take a closer look at the **entity-relationship (E-R)** and **object-oriented** models.

The E-R Model

The entity-relationship model is based on a perception of the world as consisting of a collection of basic **objects** (entities) and **relationships** among these objects.

- An **entity** is a distinguishable object that exists.
- Each entity has associated with it a set of **attributes** describing it.
- *For example,* number *and* balance *for an account entity.*
- A **relationship** is an association among several entities.
- *For example, A* cust_acct *relationship associates a customer with each account he or she has.*
- The set of all entities or relationships of the same type is called the **entity set** or **relationship set**.
- Another essential element of the E-R diagram is the **mapping cardinalities**, which express the number of entities to which another entity can be associated via a relationship set.

We'll see later how well this model works to describe real world situations.

The overall logical structure of a database can be expressed graphically by an **E-R diagram:**

- **Rectangles:** represent entity sets.
- **Ellipses:** represent attributes.
- **Diamonds:** represent relationships among entity sets.
- **Lines:** link attributes to entity sets and entity sets to relationships. See **Figure 3.3** for an example.

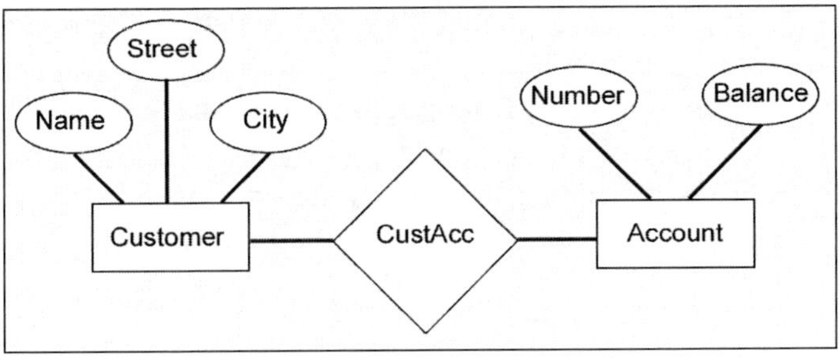

Fig. 3.3: A sample E-R diagram

The Object-oriented Model

The object-oriented model is based on a collection of objects, like the E-R model.

- An object contains values stored in **instance variables** within the object.
- Unlike the record-oriented models, these values are themselves objects.
- Thus objects contain objects to an arbitrarily deep level of nesting.
- An object also contains bodies of code that operate on the object.
- These bodies of code are called **methods**.
- Objects that contain the same types of values and the same methods are grouped into **classes**.
- A class may be viewed as a type definition for objects.
- The only way in which one object can access the data of another object is by invoking the method of that other object.
- This is called **sending a message** to the object.
- Internal parts of the object, the instance variables and method code, are not visible externally.
- Result is two levels of data abstraction.

For example, consider an object representing a bank account.

- The object contains instance variables *number* and *balance*.
- The object contains a method *pay-interest* which adds interest to the balance.
- Under most data models, changing the interest rate entails changing code in application programs.
- In the object-oriented model, this only entails a change within the *pay-interest* method.

Unlike entities in the E-R model, each object has its own unique identity, independent of the values it contains:

- Two objects containing the same values are distinct.
- Distinction is created and maintained in physical level by assigning distinct object identifiers.

Record-based Logical Models

Record-based logical models:

- Also describe data at the conceptual and view levels.
- Unlike object-oriented models, are used to
  - Specify overall logical structure of the database and
  - Provide a higher-level description of the implementation.
- Named so because the database is structured in fixed-format records of several types.
- Each record type defines a fixed number of fields or attributes.
- Each field is usually of a fixed length (this simplifies the implementation).
- Record-based models do not include a mechanism for direct representation of code in the database.
- Separate languages associated with the model are used to express database queries and updates.
- The three most widely-accepted models are the **relational, network** and **hierarchical**.

The Relational Model

- Data and relationships are represented by a collection of **tables**.
- Each **table** has a number of columns with unique names, e.g. *customer, account*.
- **Table 3.2** shows a sample relational database.

Table 3.2: A sample relational database

Name	Street	City	Number
Lowery	Maple	Queens	900
Shiver	North	Bronx	556
Shiver	North	Bronx	647
Hodges	Sidehill	Brooklyn	801
Hodges	Sidehill	Brooklyn	647

Number	Balance
900	55
556	10000
647	12345
801	9887

The Network Model

- Data are represented by collections of records.
- Relationships among data are represented by links.
- Organization is that of an **arbitrary graph**.
- **Figure 3.4** shows a sample network database that is the equivalent of the relational database of Table 3.2.

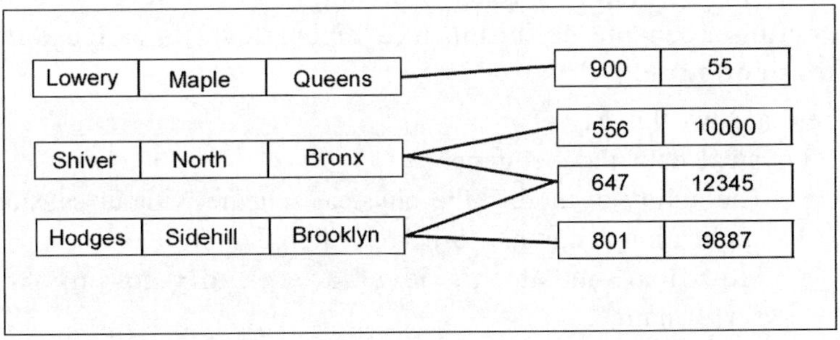

Fig. 3.4: A sample network database

The Hierarchical Model

- Similar to the network model.
- Organization of the records is as a collection of **trees**, rather than arbitrary graphs.
- **Figure 3.5** shows a sample hierarchical database that is the equivalent of the relational database of **Table 3.2**.

The relational model does not use pointers or links, but relates records by the values they contain. This allows a formal mathematical foundation to be defined.

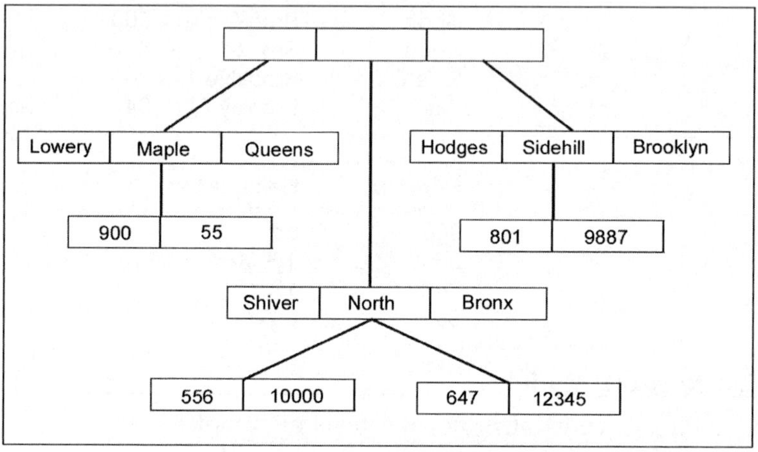

Fig. 3.5: A sample hierarchical database

DATA INDEPENDENCE

The ability to modify a scheme definition in one level without affecting a scheme definition in a higher level is called **data independence**.

There are two kinds:

1. Physical data independence
   - The ability to modify the physical scheme without causing application programs to be rewritten
   - Modifications at this level are usually to improve performance.
2. Logical data independence
   - The ability to modify the conceptual scheme without causing application programs to be rewritten.
   - Usually done when logical structure of database is altered.

NOTE: Logical data independence is harder to achieve as the application programs are usually heavily dependent on the logical structure of the data. An analogy is made to abstract data types in programming languages.

Data Definition Language (DDL)

1. Used to specify a database scheme as a set of definitions expressed in a DDL.
2. DDL statements are compiled, resulting in a set of tables stored in a special file called a **data dictionary** or **data directory**.
3. The data directory contains **metadata** (data about data)
4. The storage structure and access methods used by the database system are specified by a set of definitions in a special type of DDL called a **data storage and definition** language.
5. **Basic idea:** hide implementation details of the database schemes from the users.

Data Manipulation Language (DML)

1. **Data manipulation** is:
    - **Retrieval** of information from the database
    - **Insertion** of new information into the database
    - **Deletion** of information in the database
    - **Modification** of information in the database
2. A DML is a language which enables users to access and manipulate data. The goal is to provide efficient human interaction with the system.
3. There are two types of DML:
    - **Procedural:** the user specifies *what* data is needed and *how* to get it
    - **Nonprocedural:** the user only specifies *what* data is needed
        - Easier for user
        - May not generate code as efficient as that produced by procedural languages.
4. A **query language** is a portion of a DML involving information retrieval only. The terms DML and query language are often used synonymously.

Database Manager (For Advanced Knowledge Only)

1. The **database manager** is a **program module** which provides the interface between the low-level data stored in the database and the application programs and queries submitted to the system.

2. Databases typically require lots of storage space (gigabytes). This must be stored on disks. Data is moved between disk and main memory (MM) as needed.
3. The goal of the database system is to **simplify** and **facilitate** access to data. Performance is important. Views provide simplification.
4. **So** the database manager module is responsible for:
   - **Interaction with the file manager:** Storing raw data on disk using the file system usually provided by a conventional operating system. The database manager must translate DML statements into low-level file system commands (for storing, retrieving and updating data in the database).
   - **Integrity enforcement:** Checking that updates in the database do not violate consistency constraints (e.g. no bank account balance below $25).
   - **Security enforcement:** Ensuring that users only have access to information they are permitted to see.
   - **Backup and recovery:** Detecting failures due to power failure, disk crash, software errors, etc. and restoring the database to its state before the failure.
   - **Concurrency control:** Preserving data consistency when there are concurrent users.
5. Some small database systems may miss some of these features, resulting in simpler database managers. (For example, no concurrency is required on a PC running MS-DOS.) These features are necessary on larger systems.

Database Administrator

1. The **database administrator** is a **person** having central control over data and programs accessing that data. Duties of the database administrator include:
   - **Scheme definition:** The creation of the original database scheme. This involves writing a set of definitions in a DDL (data storage and definition language), compiled by the DDL compiler into a set of tables stored in the data dictionary.

- **Storage structure and access method definition:** Writing a set of definitions translated by the data storage and definition language compiler.
- **Scheme and physical organization modification:** writing a set of definitions used by the DDL compiler to generate modifications to appropriate internal system tables (e.g. data dictionary). This is done rarely, but sometimes the database scheme or physical organization must be modified.
- **Granting of authorization for data access:** granting different types of authorization for data access to various users
- **Integrity constraint specification:** generating integrity constraints. These are consulted by the database manager module whenever updates occur.

Database Users (For Advanced Knowledge Only)

1. The **database users** fall into several categories:
    - **Application programmers** are computer professionals interacting with the system through DML calls embedded in a program written in a host language (e.g. C, C++, Pascal).
        - These programs are called **application programs**.
        - The **DML precompiler** converts DML calls (prefaced by a special character like $, #, etc.) to normal procedure calls in a host language.
        - The host language compiler then generates the object code.
        - Some special types of programming languages combine Pascal-like control structures with control structures for the manipulation of a database.
        - These are sometimes called **fourth-generation languages**.
        - They often include features to help generate forms and display data.
    - **Sophisticated users** interact with the system without writing programs.

- They form requests by writing queries in a database query language.
- These are submitted to a **query processor** that breaks a DML statement down into instructions for the database manager module.

- **Specialized users** are sophisticated users writing special database application programs. These may be CADD systems, knowledge-based and expert systems, complex data systems (audio/video), etc.
- **Naive users** are unsophisticated users who interact with the system by using permanent application programs (e.g. automated teller machine).

Overall System Structure (For Advanced Knowledge Only)

Database systems are partitioned into modules for different functions. Some functions (e.g. file systems) may be provided by the operating system.

Components include (Refer to **Fig. 3.6**):

- **File manager** manages allocation of disk space and data structures used to represent information on disk.
- **Database manager:** The interface between low-level data and application programs and queries.
- **Query processor** translates statements in a query language into low-level instructions the database manager understands. (May also attempt to find an equivalent but more efficient form.)
- **DML precompiler** converts DML statements embedded in an application program to normal procedure calls in a host language. The precompiler interacts with the query processor.
- **DDL compiler** converts DDL statements to a set of tables containing metadata stored in a data dictionary.

DATA DICTIONARY

In addition, several data structures are required for physical system implementation:

- **Data files:** Store the database itself.

- **Data dictionary:** Stores information about the structure of the database. It is used **heavily**. Great emphasis should be placed on developing a good design and efficient implementation of the dictionary.
- **Indices:** Provide fast access to data items holding particular values.

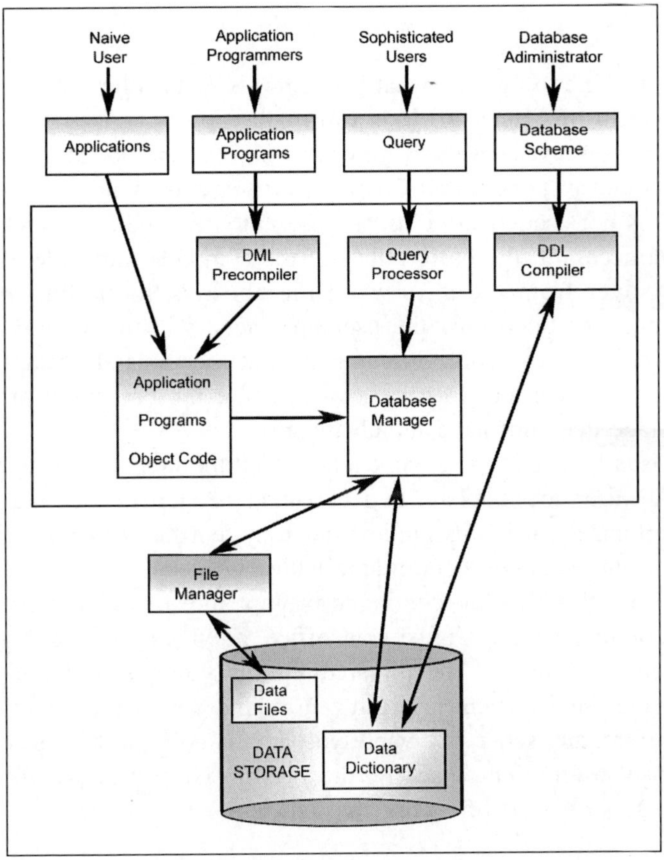

Fig. 3.6: Database system structure

Four

Introduction to Windows

Now its time to find out what Bill Gates is famous for! Welcome to the world of **Microsoft Windows**!

Windows was developed to work with the DOS operating system (described in the Second Chapter). The environment provided by DOS is not user-friendly. Its purpose is to give the user quick and direct access to the basic utility of the computer and little else; a carry-over from the days when the abilities/limitations of the computer dictated how the user interfaced with it. All tasks are accomplished by typing in commands at a command prompt (the cursor). This is not to say, however, that the command prompt interface does not have its advantages.

Usually, users or network administrators alter their system so that the user does not have to deal with this command line interface. Unfortunately, it is this kind of menu system that can prevent the user from becoming comfortable with DOS itself.

In DOS and other command-prompt interfaces, it is easy to become disoriented. Unlike your office, in which you know where you are because of the physical things you see and feel, the computer environment is organized around your work: your files. Therefore, any sense of "where you are" is going to be a sense of where you are with respect to the files on your disk. We will see how DOS organizes files later in this class.

WHAT IS MICROSOFT WINDOWS?

Windows is just a pretty interface given to DOS. What Windows does is provide the user with a few more clues about the working environment and an intuitive way of working with the files. Icons, which feign a two dimensional physical space, along with a **mouse** [*a tool used to move around the Windowing space*] make files something tangible. Like something you can "lay your hands on" (approaching the office paradigm). This, of course, is not to say that the user cannot become disoriented or that the Windows interface is entirely intuitive, its just easier to use. Thus, it makes computing more ***USER-FRIENDLY***.

STARTING MICROSOFT WINDOWS

Starting Microsoft Windows will vary depending on what computer you are using. While in most computer these days, it is pre-installed. So as soon as you switch on the computer, you enter the Windows environment. However, on your own computer in your office or at your home, you may not have this luxury (very rare). In that case, to start windows from a DOS prompt type win (as below).

c:\>win [return]

The Windows logo will briefly appear, followed by an hourglass [*symbolic of the need for you to wait patiently while Windows completes the processing of your request*] and finally the Windows **Program Manager** (which manages your software) will appear. A single headed arrow will also be visible on the screen, this is

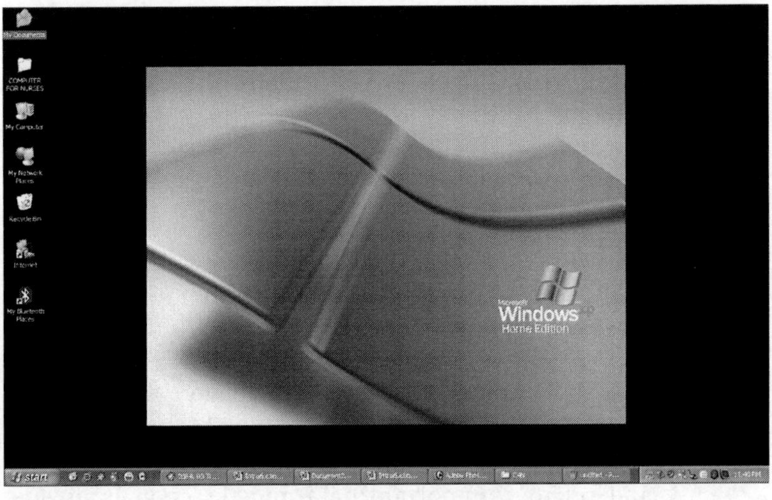

Fig. 4.1. Windows XP desktop

your **mouse pointer** [*this is an indicator of where in your workspace the mouse is located.*]

Figure 4.1 shows what the screen would look like.

WINDOWS DESKTOP

The taskbar (refer to **Fig. 4.2A**) is usually located on the bottom of the desktop. The Start button, active program buttons and the system tray are located on the taskbar.

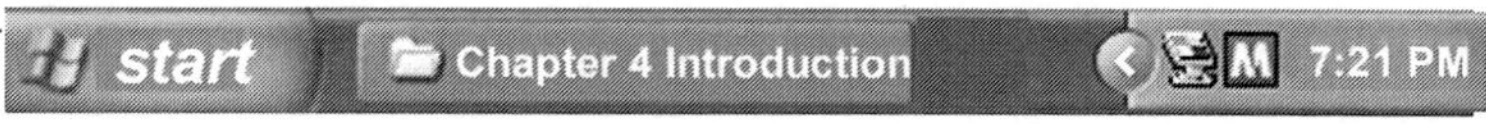

Fig. 4.2A: Taskbar

You'll typically find the System Tray in the lower right hand corner of the Windows Desktop. The system tray contains a display of the current computer time and the icons representing the programs activated when Windows first starts up.

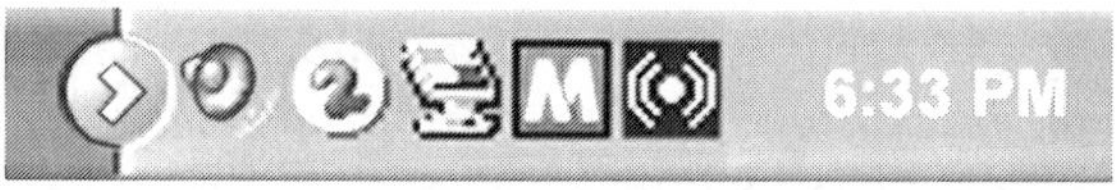

Fig. 4.2B: System tray

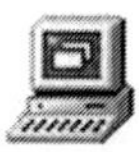

Fig. 4.2C

"My Computer" icon provides access to the different parts on your computer. You can access the different drives (hard drive, floppy drive, network drives) inside My Computer.

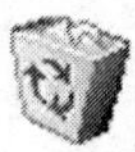

Fig. 4.2D

When you delete an object, Windows sends it to the Recycle Bin. You can restore objects that are located in the Recycle Bin or you can permanently delete them by right clicking on the Recycle Bin and select **Empty Recycle Bin**.

Fig. 4.2E

The My Documents folder is nothing more than a regular folder that resides on your Windows Desktop. However, it offers an easy-to-reach location where you can store and retrieve important data and the icon is always available in Explorer Windows and on the desktop.

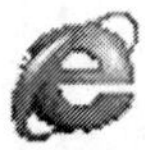

Fig. 4.2F

The Internet Explorer icon launches the Internet Explorer browser. The Internet Explorer browser is what you will use to access the Internet and the World Wide Web.

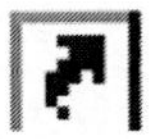

Fig. 4.2G

Icons with an arrow in the lower left corner (picture on left) are shortcut icons. If you double click on them they will open up the program that the icon displays on it.

USING THE MOUSE

The Mouse....what is this rodent for anyway??

The standard PC mouse has two buttons. To begin familiarizing yourself with the mouse, place your hand on the mouse and leaving the mouse on the desktop, move it around in a circle. You should notice that the white arrow on the screen moves in the same direction that you move the mouse. This white arrow is called a **cursor** or **mouse pointer**.

There are three ways to use the mouse button to perform a task: single clicking, double clicking and dragging. Each has a specific use and all are independent of one another.

Once you understand how to single click, double click and drag, you will be able to perform nearly every function in Windows.

CLICKING

Single Clicking

Single clicking is used to select an item or to tell the computer the item you want to work with. Items that you would normally single click on are the menu bar, any type of button and icons. Here is an example of a single clicking task:

Move the cursor so that the arrow point is resting on the word "Help" on the menu bar of any program.

Click the left mouse button once (You should notice that a menu has appeared below the word window in the menu bar).

Move the mouse to the word "About us" in the menu that you just activated.

Click the left mouse button once on the word 'About Us'. You should notice that a window has appeared with the Title "About Us (name of the program)". See **Figure 4.3**.

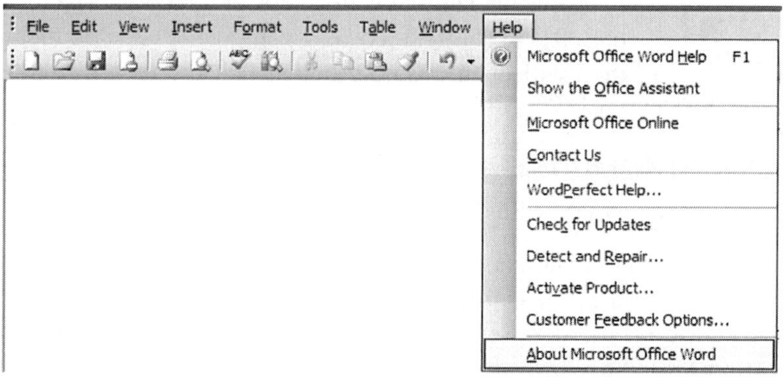

Fig. 4.3: Single Clicking

What you have just done is use single clicking to perform the task of opening a window. Let's use single clicking to close this window.

1. Move the cursor so that the point is resting above the control-menu box. Place it on 'File'.
2. Click the left mouse button once (you should notice that a menu has appeared).
3. Select "Exit" from the menu that you just activated. (This is, generally, the last item in the drop down list).
4. Or the shortcut can be adopted. If you look at the upper right corner of your screen, you will be able to see a set of buttons as shown in **Figure 4.4**.

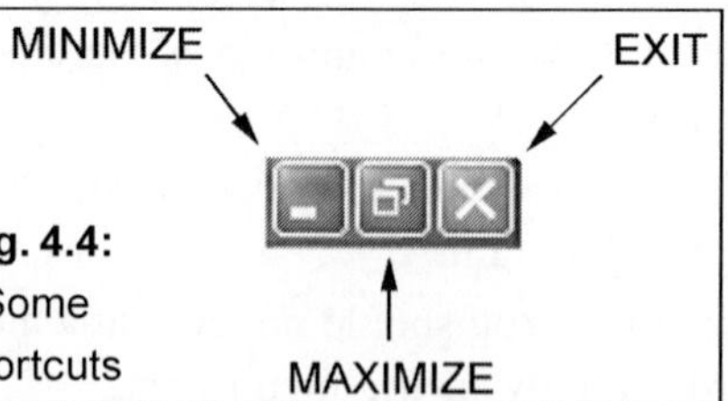

Fig. 4.4: Some shortcuts

5. By left clicking on the 'cross' (labelled EXIT), you can close the program.

Maximize a Window

1. Make the window active by clicking anywhere on it.
2. Position the pointer on the Maximize button (the center button in **Fig. 4.3**) and click the left mouse button. The window now fills your entire desktop.

Minimize a Window

1. Make the window active by clicking anywhere on it.
2. Position the pointer on the Minimize button and click the left mouse button. (the minimize button is the one in the upper right-hand side of the active window with the inverted triangle in the middle as shown in **Fig. 4.3**) The window has now turned into an Icon at the bottom of your desktop.

Now that we have mastered single clicking, let's move on to double clicking.

Double Clicking

Double clicking is a technique used to perform many tasks. While single clicking only tells the computer that the item clicked on is the one we want to use, double clicking tells the computer that this is the item we want to use and tells it to perform a task.

Double clicking is simply clicking the left mouse button twice in a row, without moving the mouse. You can think of this like a heartbeat, where two beats occur in succession.

Dragging

Dragging is a technique used to move windows and icons to different locations and also to reshape windows. This is useful to reorganize icons and windows.

In order to perform a drag, you need simply to place to cursor on the item you want to move or resize, then **hold down the left mouse button and while keeping the mouse button depressed, move the cursor** (and the item will automatically follow) to the desired location.

1. Hold down the left mouse button.
2. While holding the mouse button, move the mouse down and release the button when the window is in the desired location.

NOTE: This task can be done with any window or icon.

The other use for dragging is to reshape windows. In order to change the shape of the window, we can use the window frame (See circle in **Fig. 4.5** for the location of the window frame). We must be aware that when resizing windows, in the process we may make the window too small to see all of its contents. This is where the scroll bars will come into play. This example will make a window smaller and then we can use the scroll bars to view the parts that are to large to fit in the viewing frame.

1. Move the mouse to the bottom right corner of the window until it is directly above the window frame. You will know the cursor is in the correct position because it will turn into a double-headed arrow.
2. Hold down the left mouse button.
3. While holding down the button, move the mouse to the left until the outline of the Program Manager forms a square instead of a rectangle.
4. Release the mouse button.

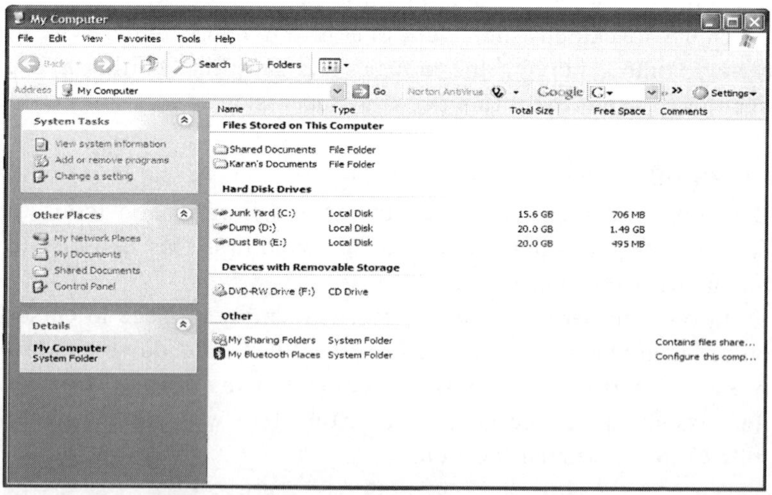

Fig. 4.5: Effect of clicking "My computer".

You should notice that the shape of the window has changed. Since we have changed the size, we cannot see all of the contents as we could before. Also, a scroll bar has appeared at the bottom of the Program Manager window. It is with this scroll bar that we can see the rest of the window.

1. Move the cursor to the right pointed arrow in the horizontal scroll bar at the bottom of the window.
2. Begin clicking the mouse button (you will notice that the icons in the Program Manager window are moving to the left and we are beginning to see the icons that we could not see a minute ago).
3. Continue to click the mouse button until the screen will not scroll any more.

We have just learned the technique of scrolling. This technique is used often, especially if you use a Windows word processor.

NOTE: If you do not adjust the scroll bars prior to resizing the window, you may not see all the icons. This is OK as you can just use the scroll bars to view them.

We have now learned the three techniques for using the mouse to navigate through Windows.

Configuration

Inside the main program group are a number of icons which relate to configuration. The most central to configuration, however, is the Control Panel program item.

Control Panel

Control Panel is full of specialized tools that are used to change the way Windows looks and behaves.

Some of these tools help you adjust settings that make your computer more fun to use. For example, use Mouse to replace standard mouse pointers with animated icons that move on your screen or use Sounds and Audio Devices to replace standard system sounds with sounds you choose. Other tools help you set up Windows so that your computer is easier to use. For example, if you are left-handed, you can use Mouse to switch the mouse buttons so that the button on the right performs the primary functions of selecting and dragging.

Although Windows still requires the files such as config.sys, autoexec.bat and others, many configurations can be made relatively easily right in the Control Panel (inside the main program group).

Opening any of these control panels (by clicking) will result in a **dialog box**. As with our previous experience with a dialog box, there are always going to be buttons and other elements to prompt you to inform Windows how to behave or look.

To activate the Control Panel, the following steps are required:

1. Click 'start' placed at the bottom left corner of your screen.
2. Go to 'settings'.
3. Click on 'Control Panel'. See **Figure 4.6**.

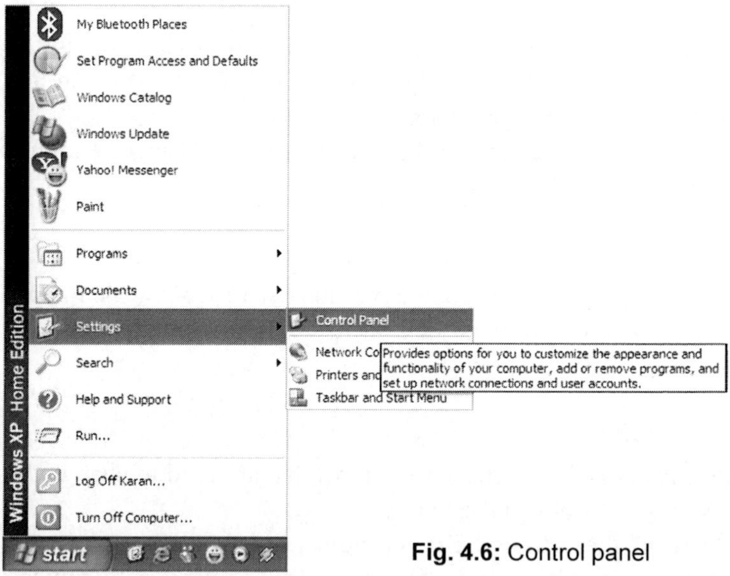

Fig. 4.6: Control panel

On following the steps described above, the Control Panel is activated. You will notice a new window with a number of icons (See **Fig. 4.7**).

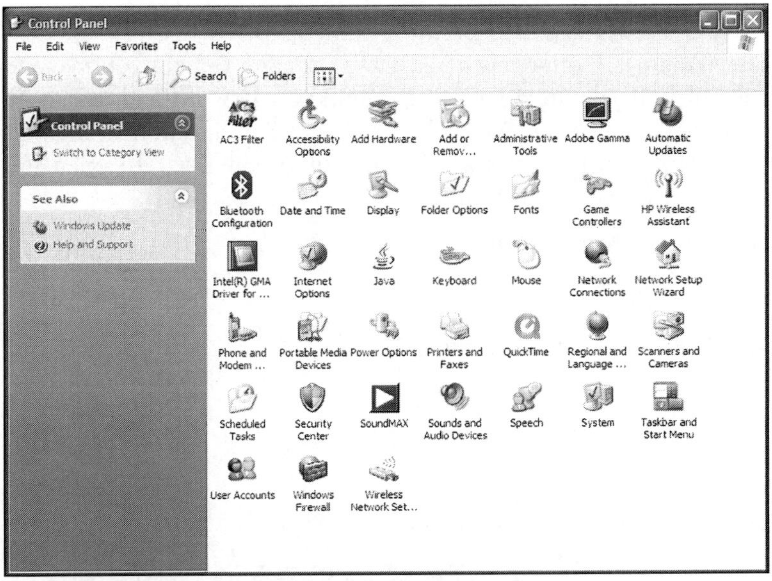

Fig. 4.7: Classic view control panel

When you first open Control Panel, you will see some of the most commonly used Control Panel items organized by category. To find out more information about an item in Control Panel while in category view, hold your mouse pointer over the icon or category name and read the text that appears. To open one of these items, click its icon or category name. Some of these items will open to a list of tasks you can perform, as well as a selection of individual Control Panel items. For example, when you click **Appearance and Themes**, you will see a list of tasks such as **Choose a screen saver** along with individual Control Panel items.

If you open Control Panel and do not see the item you want, click **Switch to Classic View**. To open an item, double-click its icon. To find out more about an item in Control Panel while in Classic Control Panel view, hold your mouse pointer over the icon and read the text that appears.

FILE MANAGEMENT

We have already learnt about the concept of files, directories and databases. Let us see how the file structure is accessed in Windows.

The Windows Explorer

The Windows Explorer is a Windows program to help you manage your files. If you are a DOS user, you know how difficult it can be to organize and keep your files up-to-date, in addition to making sure you keep a backup of all your important files. To open the Windows Explorer, perform the following steps:

Windows 98/NT/2000

1. Click on 'start'.
2. Go to 'Programs'.
3. Click on 'Windows Explorer'.

Windows XP (See **Fig. 4.8**)

1. Click on 'start'.
2. Go to 'Programs'.
3. Click on 'Accessories'.
4. Click on 'Windows Explorer'.

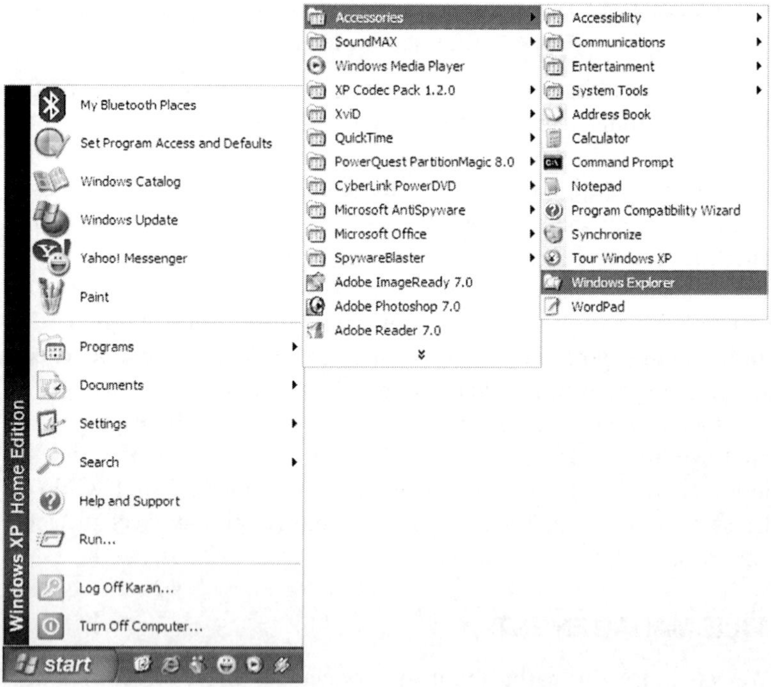

Fig. 4.8: Opening windows explorer

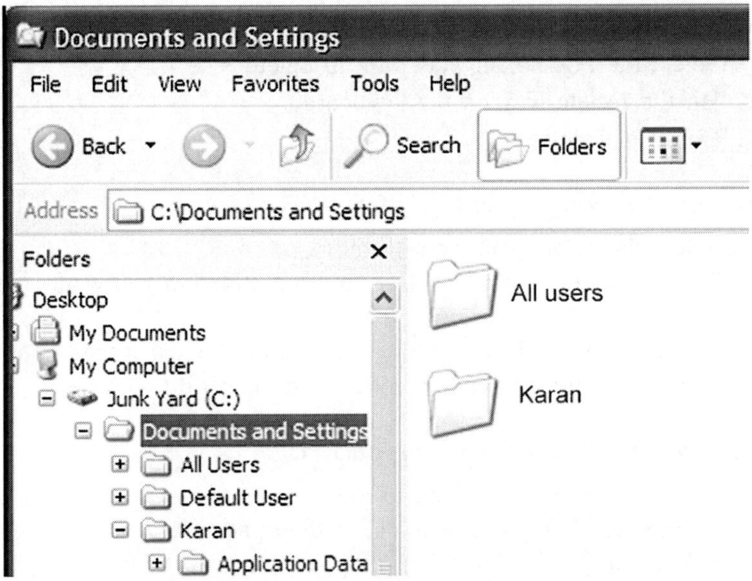

Fig. 4.9. Windows Explorer window (partial)

A Windows Explorer window similar to what you are likely to see upon opening it is shown in **Figure 4.9**.

In addition, you can now see a graphical representation of the file structure in the left pane of this window. The left window will always show directories only (represented by folder icons) and, therefore, provides a good tree diagram of the file structure of the selected disk. The right window will show you whatever is inside the directory highlighted on the left.

Also note the icons just above the split panes. These icons not only show you what disks are available to you, but what kind of disks they are:

Creating a Folder

1. Select the Drive or Folder you want to create your folder in
2. Right click in the right pane in the white area
3. Select **New**
4. Select **Folder**
5. Type in name for that folder

Deleting a File or Folder

1. Select the File/Folder you want to delete
2. Hit the Delete Key on the keyboard
3. Confirm Deletion.

Moving/Copying Files to Different Folders

1. Select the folder you want to move or copy
2. To move file — Simply drag it to the destination you want it to go to
3. To copy file — Click on Edit > Copy from the top of the screen. Then go to the destination folder and click Edit > Paste.

Copying a File/Folder to a Floppy Disk

1. Select the folder you want to move or copy
2. Right click on the file or folder in the right pane
3. Select Send To > Select 3.5 Floppy (A).

Copying a File/Folder from a Floppy Disk to other Drive

1. Select 3.5 Floppy (A:) in the left pane
2. Select the file/folder you want to copy from in the floppy drive
3. Drag it to your destination

Renaming a File or Folder

1. Select the file or folder you want to rename
2. Right click on it
3. Select Rename
4. Rename file.

Exploring File Directories

To see the contents of a particular disk, just click on its icon.

- **Click** on the "**C:**" icon.

  To display a directory, click on its icon and its contents will be displayed in the right pane.
- Click on any folder icon.

To expand a directory tree (view the subdirectories in the left window as well as the full display in the right window), simply doublclick on the folder icon of the directory you wish to expand.

Opening a Program

If the program you want to open is on the desktop, simply double-click the icon and it will open. However, if it is not located on the desktop do the following steps

1. Click on the **Start at bottom left corner of screen**
2. Click on **Programs**
3. Select the program you want to open.

Finding Files on Your Computer

If, for some reason, you cannot locate a file on your computer or home drive, you still might be able to locate it by using the Find Files Program.

1. Click on the **Start at bottom left corner of screen**
2. Click on **Find**
3. Select the **Find Files or Folders**
4. Enter your search criteria. You do not need to complete every field. Only enter the criteria you want to use for your search. Switch through the different tabs (Date, Advanced, Name and Location) to further your search
5. Click the **Find Now** button.

Locating Your Most Recent Files

Windows provides shortcuts to your most recent files, so you may get access to them very quickly.

1. Click on the **Start at bottom left corner of screen**
2. Click on **Documents**
3. Select the file that you want.

Shutting Down Windows 98

1. Click on the Start at bottom left corner of screen
2. Click on Shutdown (A Shut Down Windows dialog box will appear)

3. Click on Shut Down
4. Click on OK.

Shutting Down Windows XP

1. Click on the Start at bottom left corner of screen
2. Click on Turn Off Computer (A Shut Down Windows dialog box will appear)
3. Click on Turn Off (See **Fig. 4.10**).

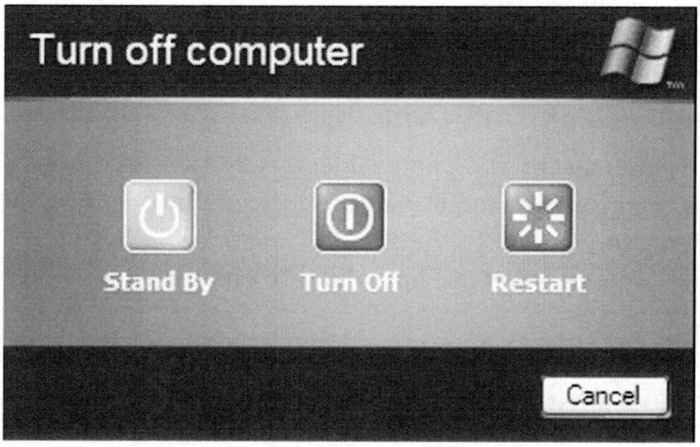

Fig. 4.10: Shutting down Windows

Restarting Windows

(To shutdown and immediately restart your computer)

1. Click on the Start at bottom left corner of screen
2. Click on Turn Off Computer (A Shut Down Windows dialog box will appear)
3. Click on Restart.

Five

Introduction to Word Processing and Microsoft Word

INTRODUCTION

There are many reasons for using computers today. Word processing is one area that has demonstrated how powerful computers can be. There are many different names of word processors. In fact today it is difficult to buy a computer without word processing software included some how. Although there are many different kinds of software, most share the same basic functions and do not require advanced computer or typing skills to use. These basic functions include:

- **Typing**
- **Saving documents**
- **Opening documents**
- **Copying**
- **Pasting**
- **Cutting**
- **Printing**
- **Checking spelling.**

Note: Most Microsoft programs allow a minimum of 3 different ways to accomplish any single task. It is not necessary for you to learn all three. Simply pick the method, which best fits your personality type.

STARTING AND QUITTING

Starting Word

1. **Start Menu:** Click on the START menu (usually the lower left-hand side of the screen) and select "Microsoft Word" from the "Programs" folder.
2. **Desktop:** (Word in the MS Office folder): Open "My Computer", open "C:", open "Programs", open "Microsoft Office" and then double click on "Microsoft Word". (See **Fig. 5.1**).

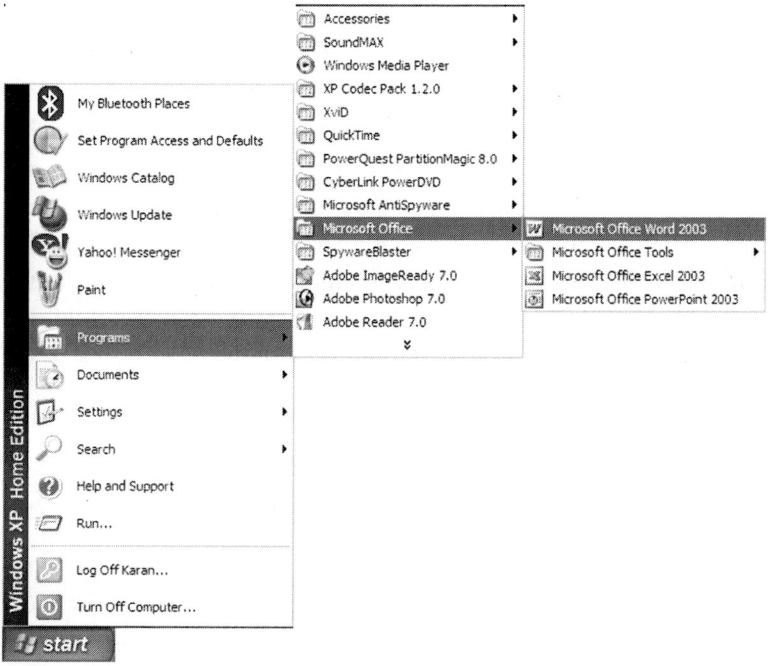

Fig. 5.1: Opening MS word

Quitting Word

- **Menu:** Go to the "File" menu and select "Exit"
- **Quit Button:** "X" button found on the upper right-hand-side of the Word window.
- **Hot Key** (Alt+F4).

Entering Text

- **Cursor-via mouse and keyboard (w and w/o Ctrl):** The cursor is the vertical line which appears on your screen and blinks. It is used to indicate where in your document you are currently editing. Clicking in the document with the left mouse button where you'd like it to be located can relocate it. Using the cursor keys can also relocate it. The cursor keys are 4 keys (located between the central keys and the numeric keypad on most keyboards) with the little arrows printed on them. Press the up arrow to move the cursor up, down arrow to go down, etc… Please note that the cursor can not be place in the middle of nowhere. It must be placed in existing text or after a "Return". If you hold down the Ctrl key while using the cursor keys, the cursor will travel up and down your text by paragraphs and left and right through your text by word.
- **Backspace:** When you press the "Backspace" key (usually found in the upper right corner of the central keys), it moves the cursor one space to the left while deleting any characters in its path.
- **Delete:** When you press the "Delete" key (usually found to the right of the "Backspace" key), you delete one character from the right of the cursor.

When **the software has loaded, it already has opened a blank document to start with. You can now start typing right away** (As illustrated in **Fig. 5.2**).

```
Dear Mom and Dad,
        I am having a geat time here on the moon. The
wether is always sunny with no clouds. The view of
the stars at night is incredible|
```

Fig. 5.2: Entering text

Since this letter is being typed using Microsoft Word from Office 97, it will underline in red any words that the software does not recognize. The red lines will not appear when printing on paper. Later in this chapter you will be shown how to use the spell checking tools.

You should also notice that the text that you are typing automatically scrolls to the next line. You do not have to hit Return or Enter at the end of each line. The only time you should hit Enter or Return is at the end of a paragraph.

- Continue to type your paragraph and hit enter or return at the end. Hit tab to indent your next paragraph and continue to type (As illustrated in **Fig. 5.3**).

```
Dear Mom and Dad,
        I am having a geat time here on the moon. The
wether is always sunny with no clouds. The view of
the stars at night is incredible. The days are always
warm, and the nights are quite chilly.
        I am having no trouble getting off the ground
here, although the small amunt of gravity does make
it difficult to build a new business. My biggest
concern will be finding  customers, even though I am
sure that sealed fresh air will be an easy item to
sell once I do|
```

Fig. 5.3: Indenting text

Saving a Document

By now it is a good idea to save your document. This is easy. Since it is the first time to save this document, click with your mouse on the word **File** at the top left hand corner of the screen. This pops up a menu. Slide down to **Save as...** and click again (Refer to **Fig. 5.4**).

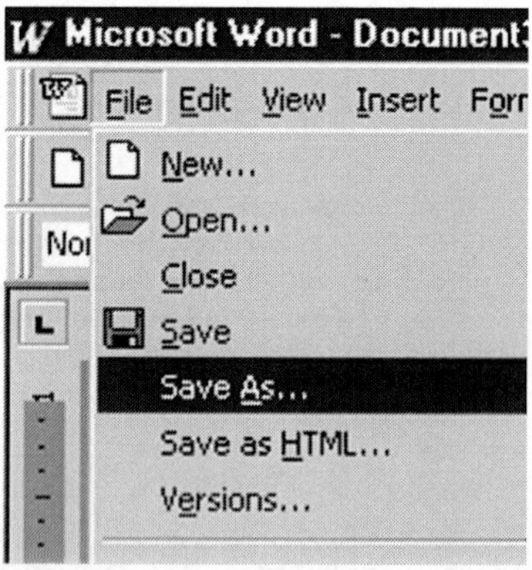

Fig. 5.4: Saving a document

A window pops up and you have to choose where you will save to. You can do this by clicking with your mouse. The example below is for Microsoft Word version 7 (Refer to **Fig. 5.5**).

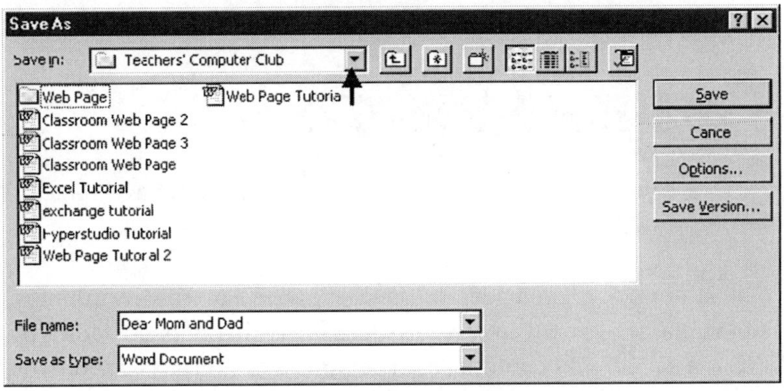

Fig. 5.5: Saving window

I am choosing to save to my "My Documents" folder. (Refer to **Fig. 5.6**).

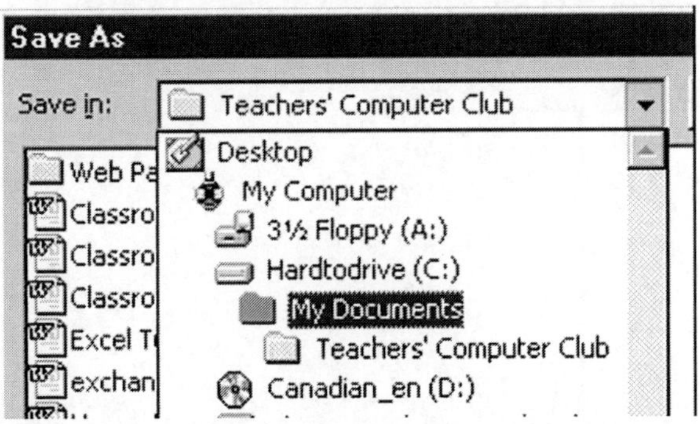

Fig. 5.6: Choosing location

Give your document a name. (Refer to **Fig. 5.7**)

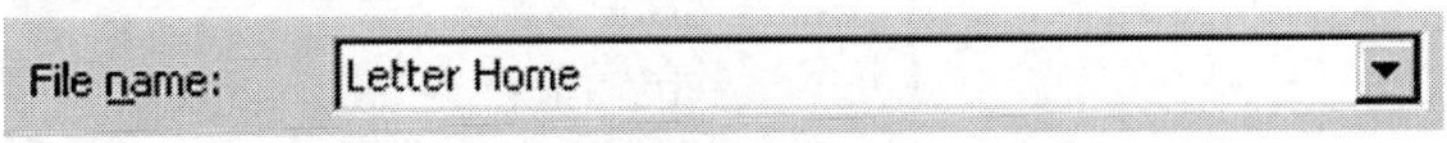

Fig. 5.7: File name

Click on save when done (Refer to **Fig. 5.8**).

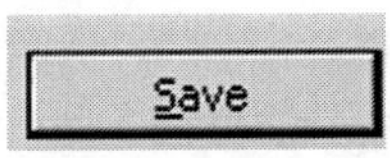

Fig. 5.8: Save button

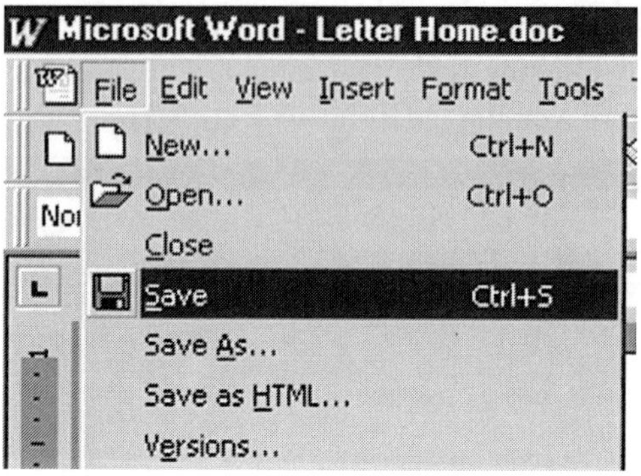

Fig. 5.9: Save from file menu

It is always a good idea to save every ten or fifteen minutes. Computers are known to *freeze* or *crash*. If this happens and you have not saved, you could lose all of your work. From now on you only need to click on **File** and slide down to **Save** (Refer to **Fig. 5.9**).

If you wish to quit and work on your document later, click on **File** and slide down to **Exit** or **Quit**. This is usually at the bottom of the File menu (Refer to **Fig. 5.10**).

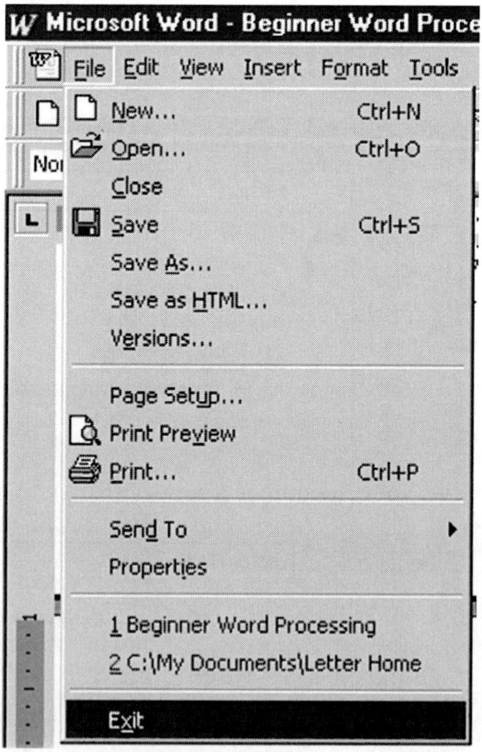

Fig. 5.10: Exiting MS WORD

Opening Your Document

Open your word processing software the same way you did in step one. Now click on the File menu again and slide down to **Open**... (Refer to **Fig. 5.11**).

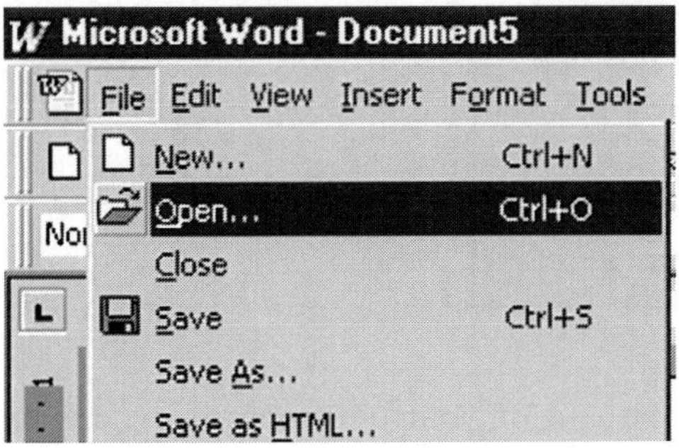

Fig. 5.11: Opening a document

Your document should now appear before you on the screen.

Copying and Pasting

If you wish to copy any part of your document to paste to another part, you first have to select the text that you want copied. This is done by *clicking and dragging* over top the text to copy. Click and hold the mouse button at the beginning of the text, then carefully *drag* it to the end of the text. All of the text you selected will appear highlighted. If you highlight too much or not enough, do not worry, just try again (Refer to **Fig. 5.12**).

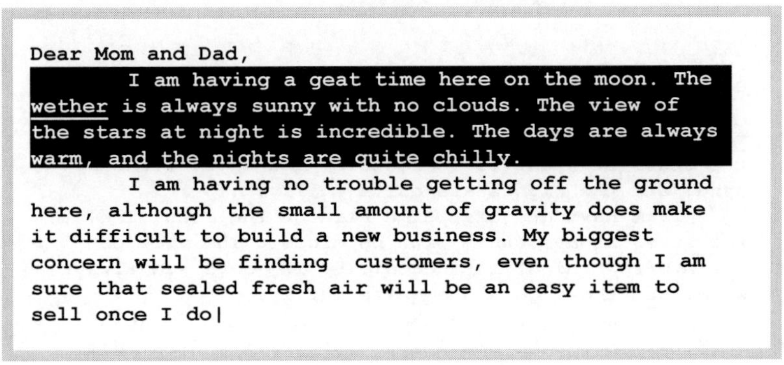

Dear Mom and Dad,

I am having a geat time here on the moon. The wether is always sunny with no clouds. The view of the stars at night is incredible. The days are always warm, and the nights are quite chilly.

I am having no trouble getting off the ground here, although the small amount of gravity does make it difficult to build a new business. My biggest concern will be finding customers, even though I am sure that sealed fresh air will be an easy item to sell once I do

Fig. 5.12: Selecting text

Click on the **Edit** menu and slide down to copy. This copies what you selected to a *virtual* clipboard which you can not see (Refer to **Fig. 5.13**).

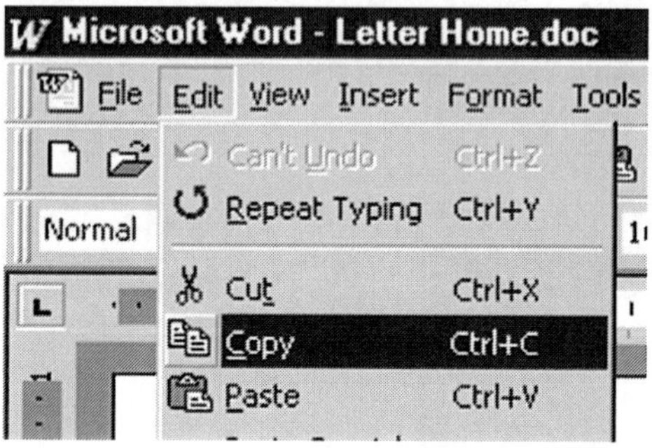

Fig. 5.13: Copying text

Click your mouse at the end of your document or wherever you want to paste to. Click on the **Edit** menu and slide down to **Paste** (Shortcut: **ctrl** + **v**) (Refer to **Fig. 5.14**).

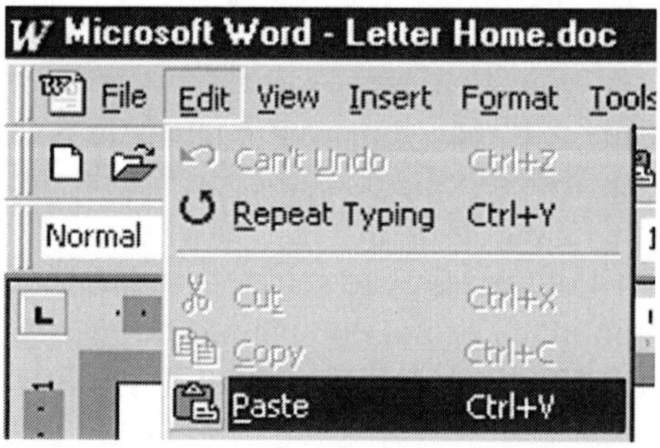

Fig. 5.14: Pasting text

The text that you copied to the *virtual* clipboard then appears right where you clicked (Refer to **Fig. 5.15**).

Dear Mom and Dad,

I am having a geat time here on the moon. The wether is always sunny with no clouds. The view of the stars at night is incredible. The days are always warm, and the nights are quite chilly.

I am having a geat time here on the moon. The wether is always sunny with no clouds. The view of the stars at night is incredible. The days are always warm, and the nights are quite chilly.

I am having no trouble getting off the ground here, although the small amunt of gravity does make

Fig. 5.15: A second copy of selected text has been pasted

Cutting and Pasting

If you wish to move some text from one place to another, you might want to cut the text instead of copying it. Cutting and copying are the same, except that cutting removes the text but still puts it on the *virtual* clipboard. To do so click and drag over the text that you want cut (Refer to **Fig. 5.16**).

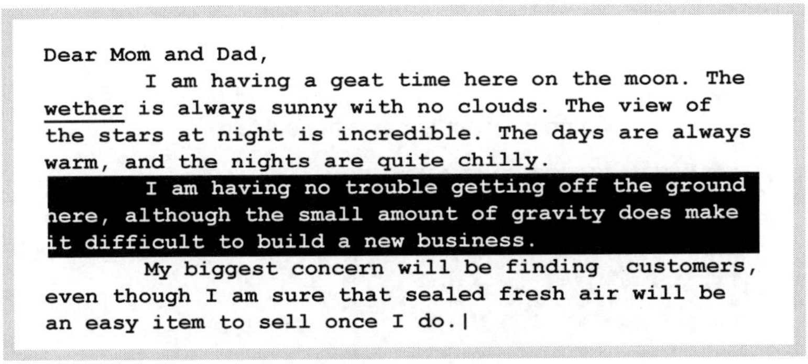
Dear Mom and Dad,

I am having a geat time here on the moon. The wether is always sunny with no clouds. The view of the stars at night is incredible. The days are always warm, and the nights are quite chilly.

I am having no trouble getting off the ground here, although the small amount of gravity does make it difficult to build a new business.

My biggest concern will be finding customers, even though I am sure that sealed fresh air will be an easy item to sell once I do.

Fig. 5.16: Selecting text you want to cut

Click on **Edit** and slide down to **Cut**. This removes the text and places it on to the invisible *virtual* clipboard (Refer to **Fig. 5.17**).

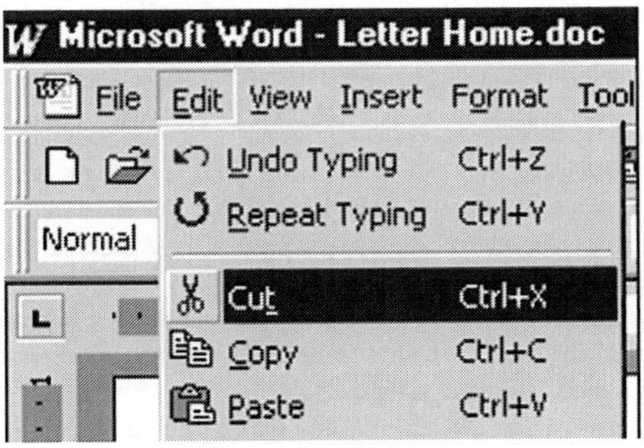

Fig. 5.17: Cutting text that was selected

Click where you want to paste the text to (Refer to **Fig. 5.18**).

Click on **Edit** and choose **Paste** (Refer to **Fig. 5.19**).

Dear Mom and Dad,
I am having a geat time here on the moon. The wether is always sunny with no clouds. The view of the stars at night is incredible. The days are always warm, and the nights are quite chilly.
My biggest concern will be finding customers, even though I am sure that sealed fresh air will be an easy item to sell once I do.

Fig. 5.18: The cut text is not seen. The pointer is positioned where we want to paste the cut text

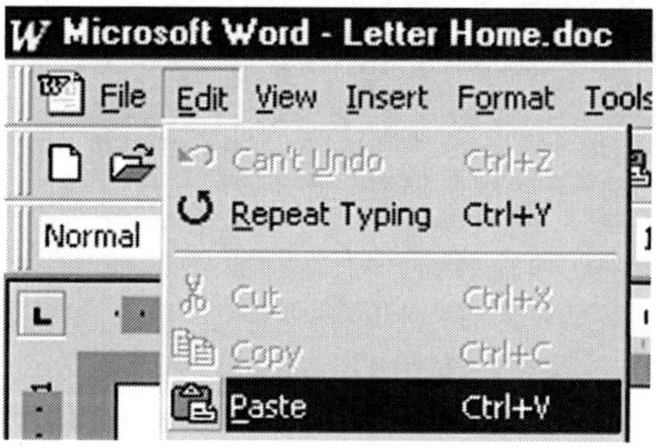

Fig. 5.19: Pasting text

The text that you copied to the *virtual* clipboard then appears right where you clicked (Refer to **Fig. 5.20**).

Dear Mom and Dad,
I am having a geat time here on the moon. The wether is always sunny with no clouds. The view of the stars at night is incredible. The days are always warm, and the nights are quite chilly.
My biggest concern will be finding customers, even though I am sure that sealed fresh air will be an easy item to sell once I do.
I am having no trouble getting off the ground here, although the small amount of gravity does make it difficult to build a new business.

Fig. 5.20: The text that had been cut has been copied at the new place

Spell Checking

The spell checker is a great tool to have on a word processor, but it is not perfect. It only looks at every word that you typed, one at a time and checks it with a dictionary. It does not look at each word in its context. Therefore if you typed *their* when you really wanted the word *there*, it will not correct the mistake. This means that you will still have to proof read your document yourself.

Unlike all of the features explained before, the spell checking tool is not in the same place for all software. It is often found in the **Edit** menu or the **Tools** menu. In this case (Microsoft Word) it is in the Tools menu. So we click on the Tools menu and slide down to **Spelling and Grammar**.... (Refer to **Fig. 5.21**).

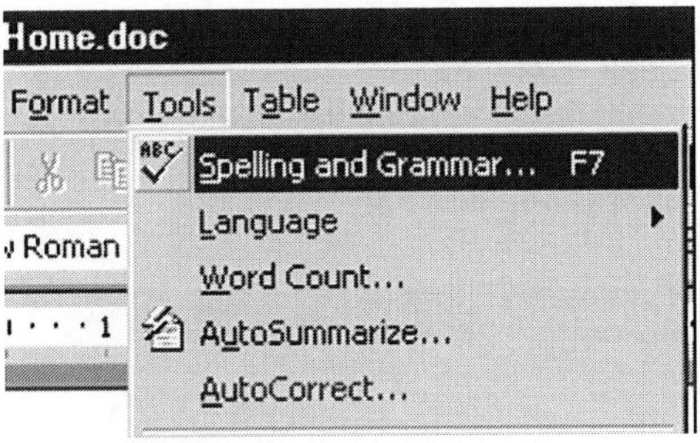

Fig. 5.21: Spelling and grammar check

A spell check window pops up. Depending upon your software, you may have to click on a button that says Start. In this case we do not have to, it starts spell checking right away. When it finds a word that it does not recognize, it will show you and also give some alternative suggestions. If the word is spelled correct (spell checking does not usually recognize names as an example) then click on **Ignore** or **Ignore All**. If it is misspelled, click on the correct word in the suggestions and then click on **Change**. Do not click on the **Add** button or in some cases the Learn button, as this will add the misspelled word to the computer's dictionary (Refer to **Fig. 5.22**).

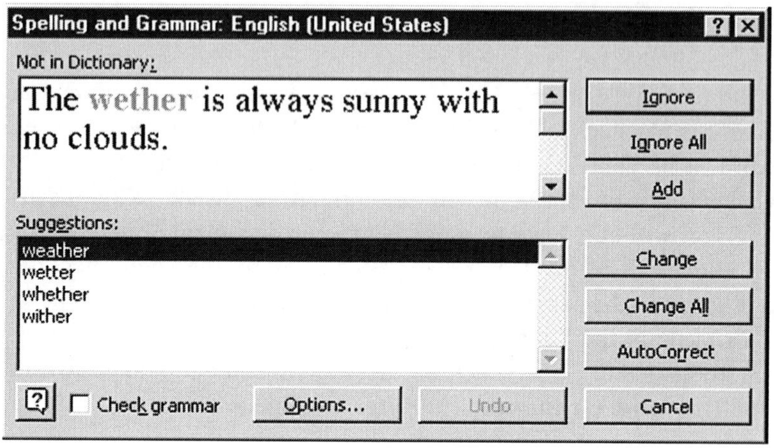

Fig. 5.22: Correcting wrong spellings

When it has finished checking all of the words you have typed, it will usually let you know. Click on **OK** or in some cases **Done** (Refer to **Fig. 5.23**).

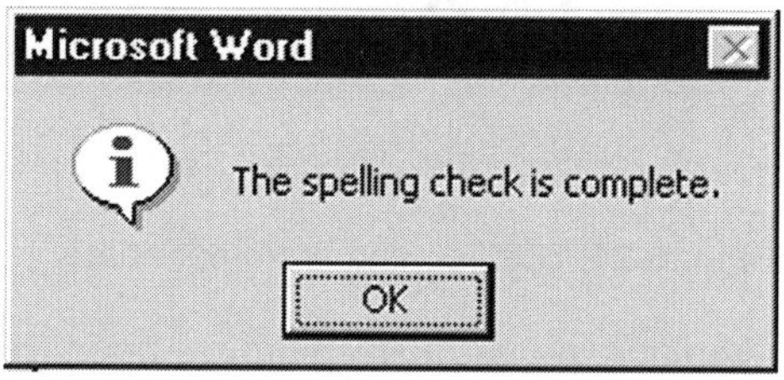
Microsoft Word
The spelling check is complete.
OK

Fig. 5.23: Program tell you that spell check is complete

Printing

Print Preview

In short, the Print Preview feature allows you to see how a document will look when you print it. It also allows you to do last minute formatting on the document (Refer to **Fig. 5.24**).

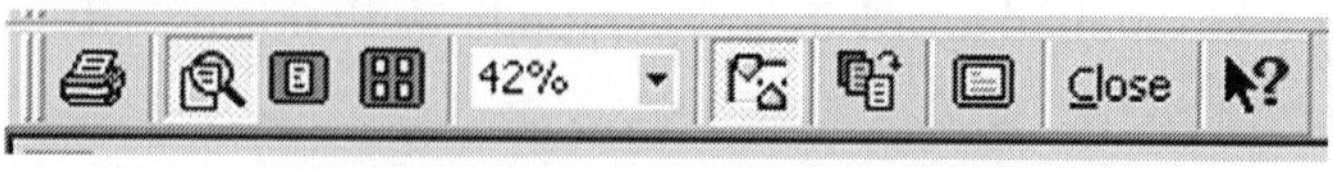
42%
Close

Fig. 5.24: Print preview toolbar

Print Preview Tools from Left to Right

- **Print:** Already explained
- **Magnify:** Allows you to zoom in on parts of the document
- **One Page:** Previews only one page at a time
- **Multiple Page:** Previews multiple pages at one time
- **Zoom Control:** How much are you zoomed in/out?
- **View Rulers:** Margins: Allows you to adjust margins from the Print Preview screen
- **Shrink to Fit:** "when one, just isn't enough": Shrinks your document to fit on one less page
- **Full Page:** Removes all toolbars from window, thus giving you more viewing real estate
- **Close:** Self explanatory
- **Help:** Self explanatory

When you have finished working on a document, and have checked it thoroughly, you will probably want to print your document. To do this click on the **File** menu and slide down to **Print** (Refer to **Fig. 5.25**).

A printing window pops up. There is a lot of information here and you probably do not need to worry about most of it. You can change the number of copies you wish to print, but otherwise just click **OK** or **Print** (Refer to **Fig. 5.26**).

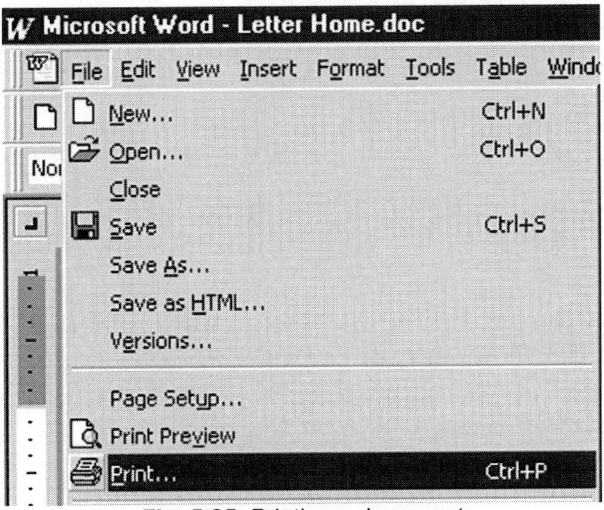

Fig. 5.25: Printing a document

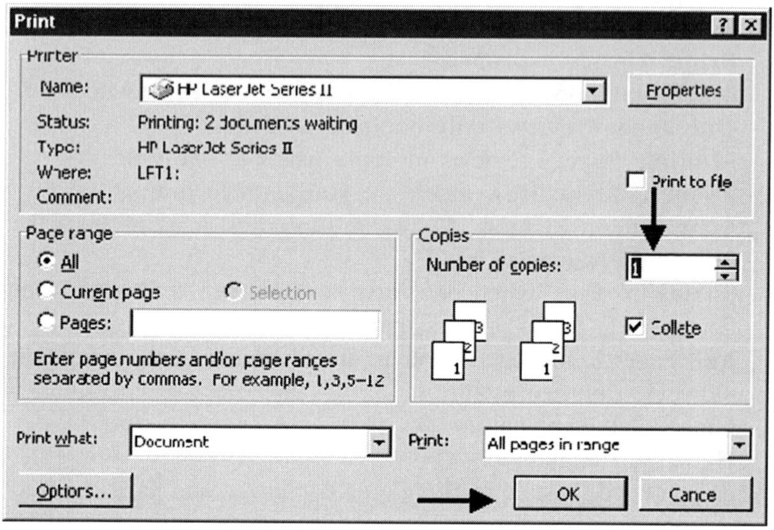

Fig. 5.26: Box to decide options for printing

UNDO - REDO

If you ever make a mistake, do not worry, just click on **Edit** and slide down to **Undo** (Refer to **Fig. 5.27**).

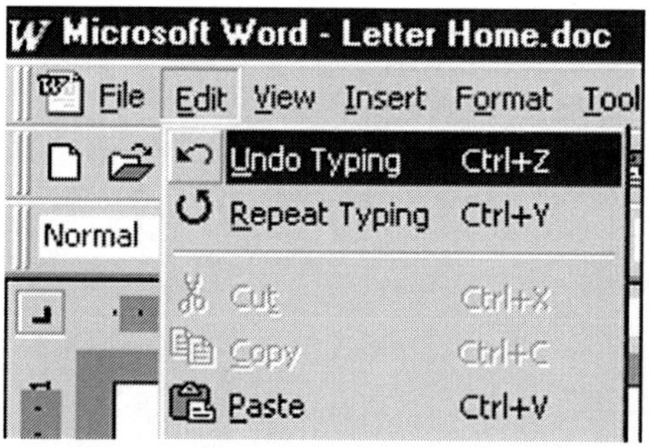

Fig. 5.27: Box to undo some wrong action

When you are finished and want to leave, save and click on **File** and slide down to **Quit** or **Exit** at the bottom of the menu.

SELECTING

The first step in editing your text, is selecting the text you wish to edit. For example, if you select nothing and then tell the computer to make your selection "bold". The computer makes "nothing" bold.

For easily selecting different amounts of text and graphics by using the mouse, see **Table 5.1**.

Table 5.1: Shortcuts for selection of text

To select	*Do this*
Any amount of text	Drag over the text.
A word	Double click the word.
A graphic	Click the graphic.
A line of text	Move the pointer to the left of the line until it changes to a right-pointing arrow and then click.
Multiple lines of text	Move the pointer to the left of the lines until it changes to a right-pointing arrow and then drag up or down.
A sentence	Hold down CTRL and then click anywhere in the sentence.
A paragraph	Move the pointer to the left of the paragraph until it changes to a right-pointing arrow and then double-click. Or triple-click anywhere in the paragraph.
Multiple paragraphs	Move the pointer to the left of the paragraphs until it changes to a right-pointing arrow and then double-click and drag up or down.
A large block of text	Click at the start of the selection, scroll to the end of the selection and then hold down SHIFT and click.
An entire document	Move the pointer to the left of any document text until it changes to a right-pointing arrow and then triple-click.

Select All: Choose "**Select All**" from the "**Edit**" menu or press the Hot Key **Ctrl+A**=Select All

Formatting Text

Font formatting: The most commonly used font formatting options are available on the "formatting" toolbar. All of the font formatting options are available when you select "Font" from either the "Format" menu or the right-button clicked mouse (Refer to **Fig. 5.28**).

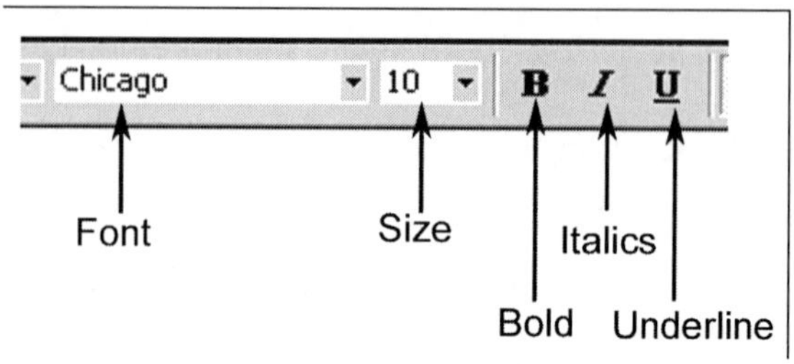

Fig. 5.28: Formatting toolbar

Fonts: The shapes of your letters.

NOTE: Different fonts will be available on different machines. If preparing a document to be viewed on different companies, you should use standardized fonts such as "Time-Roman", "Arial", etc.

Font Size: The size of the letter

Bold, Italics, Underline and Color: Self explanatory. There are also hot keys for the following: Ctrl+B=Bold, Ctrl+I=Italics, Ctrl+U=Underline (Refer to **Fig. 5.28**).

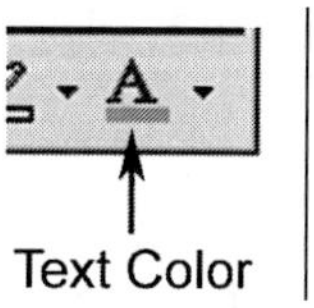

Fig. 5.29: Selecting text color

Effects (only available through Format command): These include a number of additional font formatting options such as superscript, subscript, emboss, shadow, etc.

Character spacing: (only available through Format command): Allows you adjust the amount of space between individual characters as well as their position relative to the line of text.

Animation: (Office '97 Only) (only available through Format command): These visual effects are useful only for electronic distribution. None of these effects will print out (Refer to **Fig. 5.30**).

Paragraph Formatting

The most commonly used paragraph formatting options are available on the "formatting" toolbar. All of the paragraph

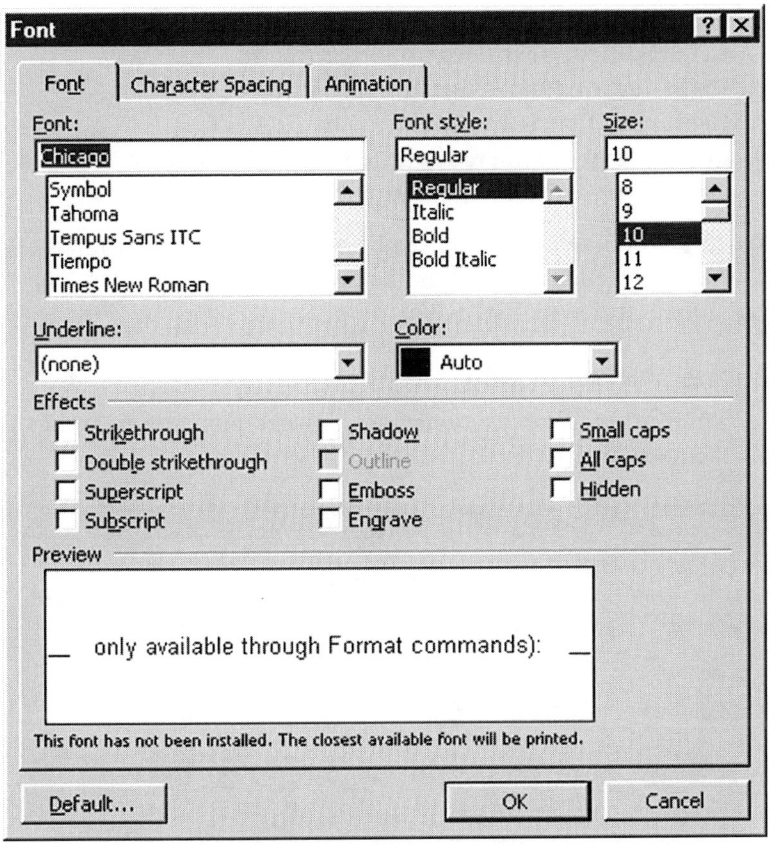

Fig. 5.30: Advanced font options

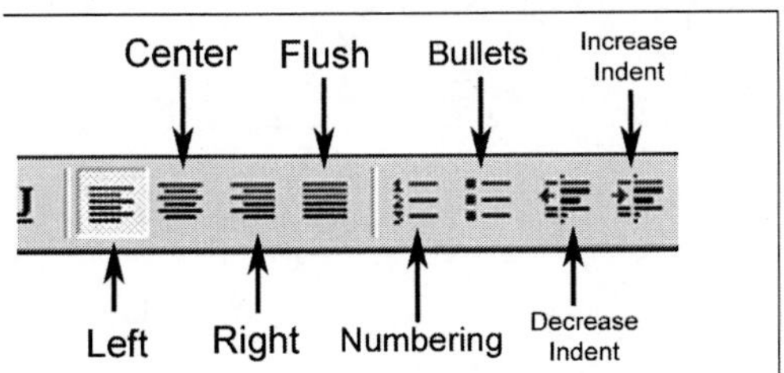

Fig. 5.31: Paragraph formatting options

formatting options are available when you select "Paragraph" from either the "Format" menu or the right-button clicked mouse (Refer to **Figure 5.31**).

Alignment: Adjusts how the text is aligned in the document.

- **Left justified:** Text lines up to the left
- **Right justified:** Text lines up to the right
- **Centered:** Text is centered
- **Flush:** Text is centered with enough spaces between words that the left and right hand extremes also line up.

Spacing: (only accessible through the Format command): Adjust the "Line Spacing" as well as the spacing before or after a new paragraph (Refer to **Fig. 5.32**).

Bullets and Numbering

- **Numbering:** Word automatically places numbers in front of each new line of text.

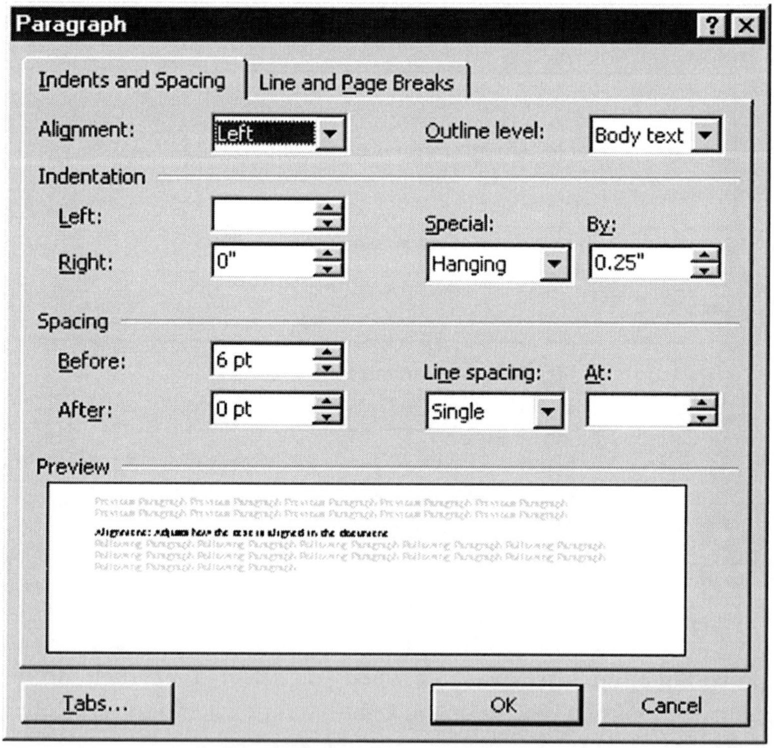

Fig. 5.32: Adjustng line spacing

- **Bullets:** Word automatically places bullets in front of each new line of text.
- **Indentation:** Increase and decrease the amount of space between the left margin and the left side of the text.
- **Bullets and Numbering format** (only accessible through the Format command): Allows you to change the style of your bullets and numbering system.

Format Painter: Once you get a section of text to look the way you want it to, you can copy all of its attributes to another section of text using the "**Format Painter**" tool. This tool looks like a paintbrush and is located to the right of the "**Paste**" tool on the standard toolbar.

Styles: Like the "Format Painter", "Styles" allow you to pass the attributes of one section of text to another. Unique to "Styles", you can create format templates such as "normal" or "headline" to apply to the appropriate sections of your document. Should you

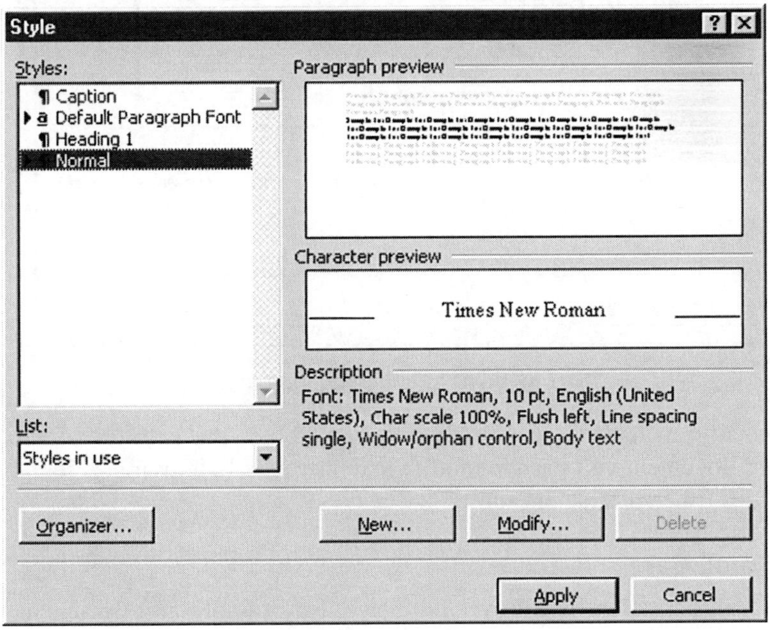

Fig. 5.33: Window showing styles

change your mind about what a "headline" looks like, simply modify the settings for that "style" and all of the sections of text which were formatted as "headline" will automatically take on the new settings (Refer to **Fig. 5.33**).

***Tabs and Margins*:** Before adjusting "Tabs and Margins", it is best to be in "Layout" view. This is accomplished by selecting "Page Layout" from the "View" menu.

- **For the whole document:** To adjust the margins for the entire document, select "Page Setup" from the "File" menu, (Refer to **Fig. 5.34**).

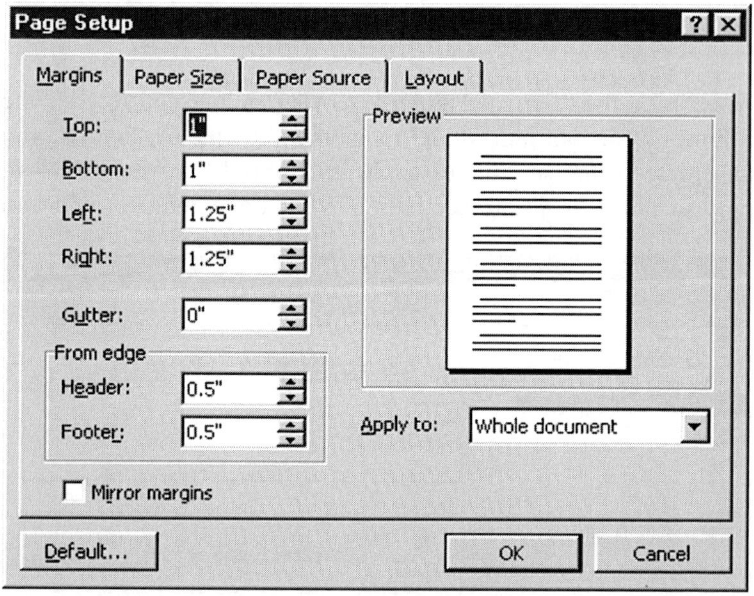

Fig. 5.34: Seting page margins

- **For a section of the document:** Select the section of the document you wish to modify and move the little triangles found on the ruler at the top of the page.

Scroll Bars

Scroll bars crop up all over the place, for example in a document, when looking for a font or font size, so it is well worth becoming familiar with the way that they work (Refer to **Fig. 5.35**).

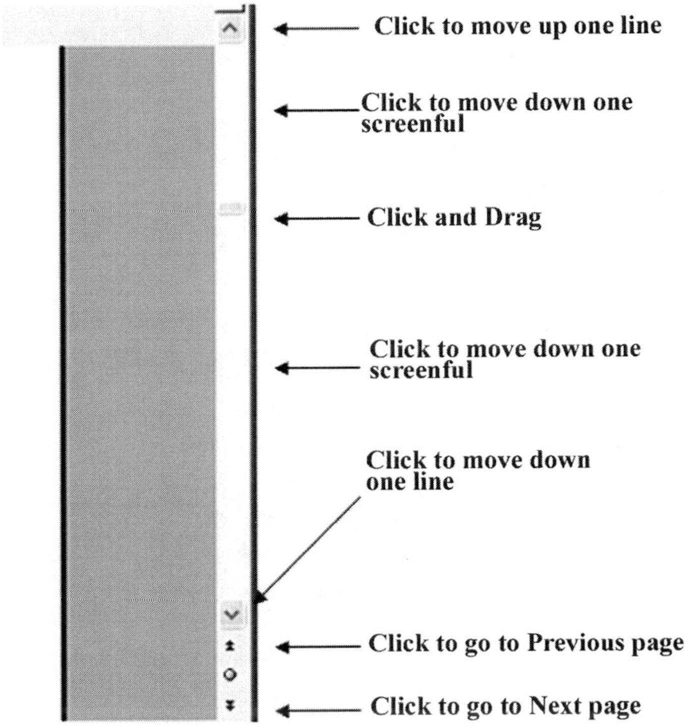

Fig. 5.35: Scrolling through text

Opening and Saving Shortcuts

New File

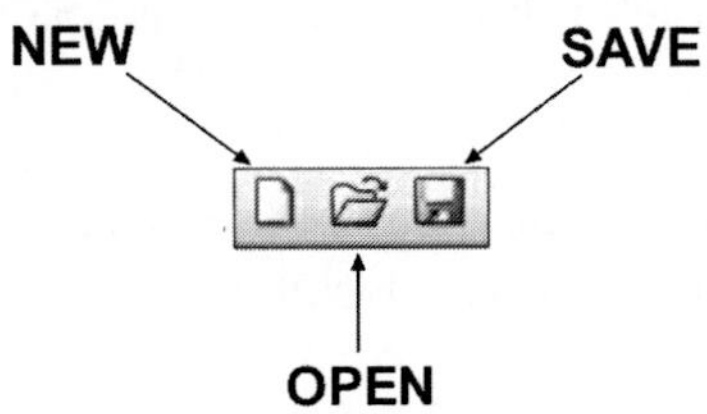

Fig 5.36: The operations can also be directly performed by clicking on the desired button

- **via Hot Key:** (Ctrl)+N
- **via Desktop:** Click on the desktop or in a folder with your *right* mouse button. Select "New" from the resulting menu and

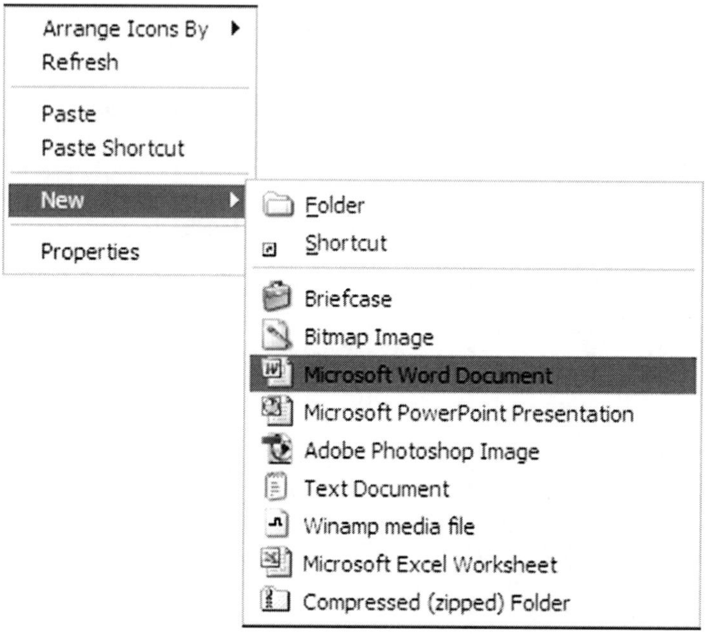

Fig. 5.37: Opening a new MS word document from the desktop

then select "Microsoft Word Document". Name the document and double-click on it to launch Word (As illustrated in **Fig. 5.37**).

Saving a File

On the PC, Word defaults to saving new files to the "My Documents" folder. Word defaults to saving a file back to where it was loaded from:

- **via Hot Key:** (Ctrl)+S
- "Save As" can be used to save a second copy of your "open" document with a new name and/or a new location.

Opening a File

- **via Hot Key:** (Ctrl)+O
- **via Desktop:** Find the file (hopefully in your Home Directory) and double click on its icon.

HELP

- All of the tools on the Word Toolbar, will identify themselves if you hold the mouse over them without pressing a button.
- Additional help can be found by selecting an option from the "Help" menu.
- Even more help can be brought online by pressing the F1 button. In Office '97, this brings up the Office Assistant who recognizes most "real language" requests.

That's it! Although there are many more things to do on word processors, these are the basics. Go ahead and practice and get used to your word processor. ***Do not be afraid to experiment a little with the other functions when you are ready.***

Six

Introduction to Microsoft Excel

INTRODUCTION

Spreadsheets are a great tool for doing math related jobs. They can save one an incredible amount of time. As professionals we are always working with numbers, whether it be calculating marks, counting money, fund raising, etc. Somebody who is comfortable with spreadsheets can avoid hours of dreary repetitive work by doing these tasks with a spreadsheet. Spreadsheets have become even more powerful and easy to use than ever before. They are extremely useful today.

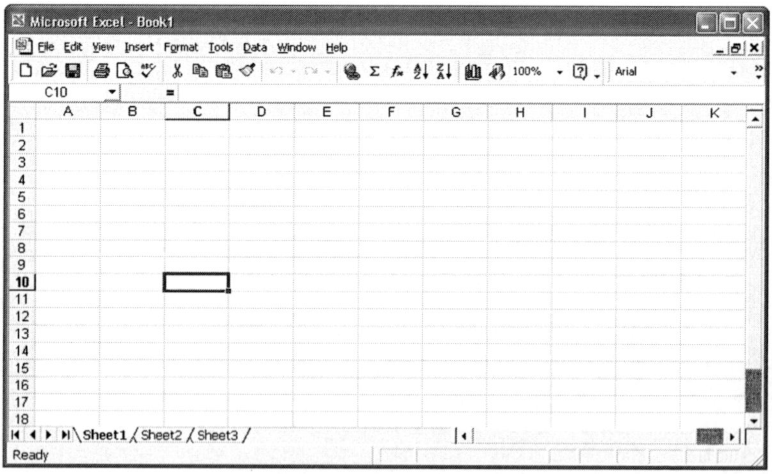

Fig. 6.1: MS Excel screen

ENTERING TEXT AND NUMBERS

The Microsoft Excel Window

This Chapter teaches Microsoft Excel basics (since it is the most commonly used spreadsheet program used these days). To begin, open Microsoft Excel. Then, if necessary, click the **X** in the upper right corner of the task pane to close the task pane.

The screen shown in **Figure 6.1** will appear.

The MS-Excel Screen

The Title Bar

This section will familiarize you with the Microsoft Excel screen. We will start with the Title bar, which is located at the very top of the screen. On the Title bar, Microsoft Excel displays the name of the workbook you are currently using. At the top of your screen, you should see "Microsoft Excel - Book1" or a similar name (**Fig. 6.2**).

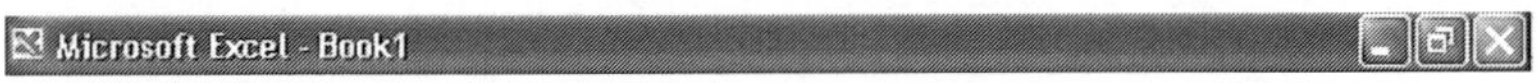

Fig. 6.2: The title bar

The Menu Bar

The Menu bar (**Fig. 6.3**) is directly below the Title bar. The menu begins with the word File and continues with Edit, View, Insert, Format, Tools, Data, Window and Help. You use a menu to give instructions to the software. Point with your mouse to a menu option and click the left mouse button. A drop-down menu opens. You can now use the left and right arrow keys on your keyboard to move left and right across the Menu bar. You can use the up and down arrow keys to move up and down the drop-down menu. To choose an option, highlight the item on the drop-down menu and press Enter. An ellipse after a menu item signifies additional options; if you choose that option, a dialog box opens.

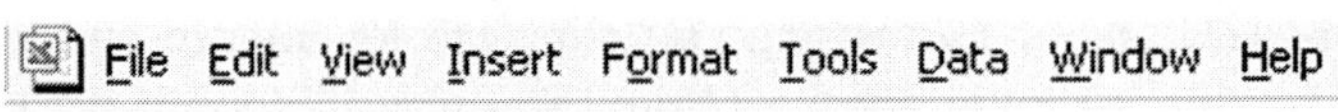

Fig. 6.3: The menu bar

Toolbars

Toolbars (**Figs 6.4 and 6.5**) provide shortcuts to menu commands. Toolbars are generally located just below the Menu bar. Before proceeding with this lesson, make sure the toolbars you will use — Standard and Formatting — are available. Follow the steps outlined here:

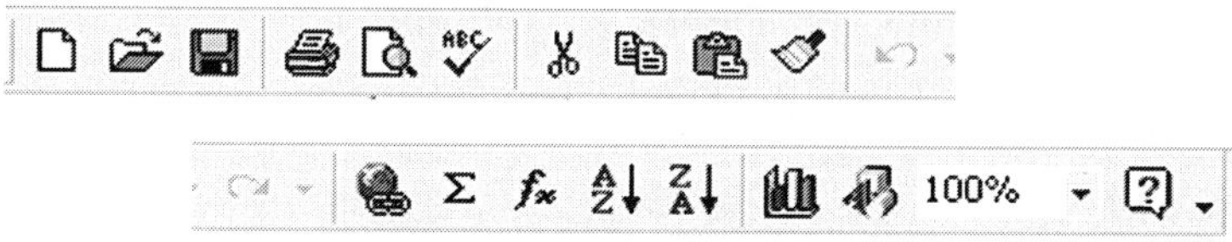

Fig. 6.4: The Standard tool bar
(shown in two parts for clarity)

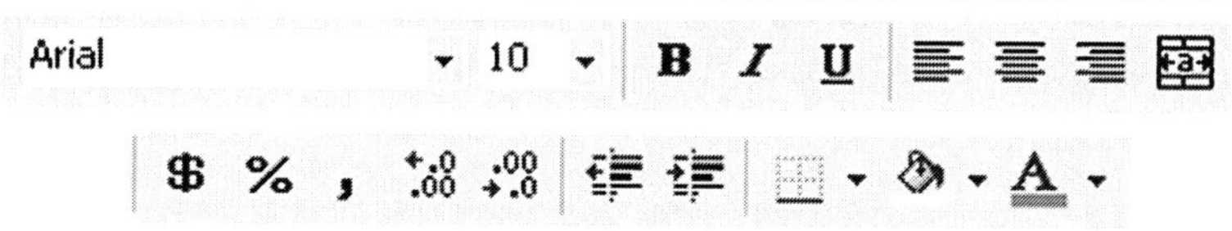

Fig. 6.5: The Formatting tool bar
(shown in two parts for clarity)

1. Point to *View*, which is located on the Menu bar.
2. Click the left mouse button.
3. Press the down arrow key until Toolbars is highlighted.
4. Press the right arrow key.
5. Both Standard and Formatting should have a check mark next to them. If both have a check mark next to them, press Esc two times to close the menu. If either does not have a check mark, press the down arrow key until Customize is highlighted.
6. Press Enter. The customize dialog box opens.
7. Choose the Toolbars tab.
8. Point to the box or boxes next to the unchecked word or words, Standard and/or Formatting and click the left mouse button. A check mark should appear. (***Note*:** You turn the check mark on and off by clicking the left mouse button).

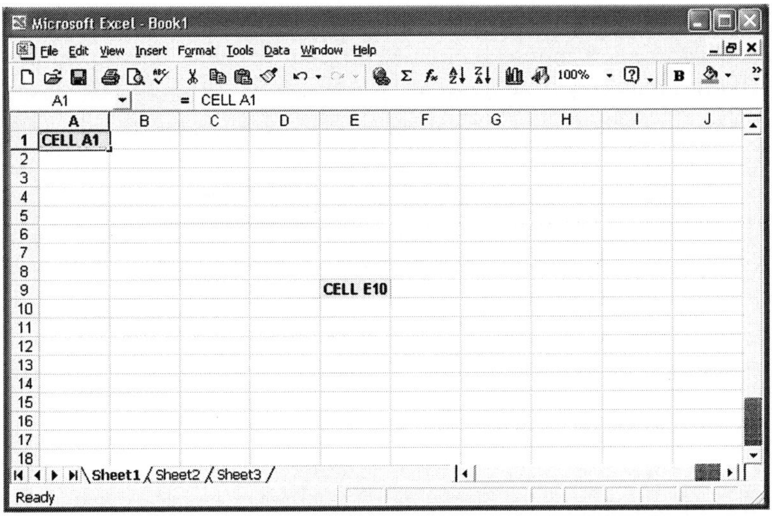

Fig. 6.6: An Excel Worksheet

9. Point to Close and click the left mouse button to close the dialog box.

Worksheets

Microsoft Excel consists of worksheets (**Fig. 6.6**). Each worksheet contains columns and rows. The columns are lettered A to IV; the rows are numbered 1 to 65536. The combination of a column coordinate and a row coordinate make up a cell address. For example, the cell located in the upper left corner of the worksheet is cell A1, meaning column A, row 1. Cell E10 is located under column E on row 10. You enter your data into the cells on the worksheet.

The Formula Bar

If the Formula bar (**Fig. 6.7**) is turned on, the cell address displays in the Name box on the left side of the Formula bar. Cell entries display on the right side of the Formula bar. Before proceeding, make sure the Formula bar is turned on.

1. Point to View, which is located on the Menu bar.
2. Click the left mouse button. A drop-down menu opens. On the drop-down menu, if Formula Bar has a check mark next to it, the Formula bar is turned on. Press the Esc key to close the drop-down menu.
3. If Formula Bar does not have a check mark next to it, press the down arrow key until Formula Bar is highlighted; then press Enter. The Formula bar should now appear below the toolbars.
4. Note that the current cell address displays on the left side of the Formula bar.

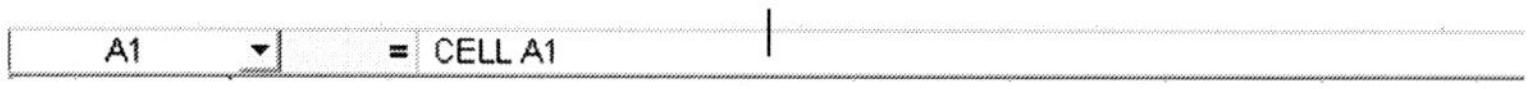

Fig. 6.7: Formula bar

The Status Bar

If the Status bar (**Fig. 6.8**) is turned on, it appears at the very bottom of the screen. Before proceeding, make sure the Status bar is turned on.

1. Point to View, which is located on the Menu bar.
2. Click the left mouse button. A drop-down menu opens.
3. On the drop-down menu, if Status Bar has a check mark next to it, it is turned on. Press the Esc key to close the drop-down menu.
4. If Status Bar does not have a check mark next to it, press the down arrow key until Status Bar is highlighted; then press Enter. The Status bar should now appear at the bottom of the screen.

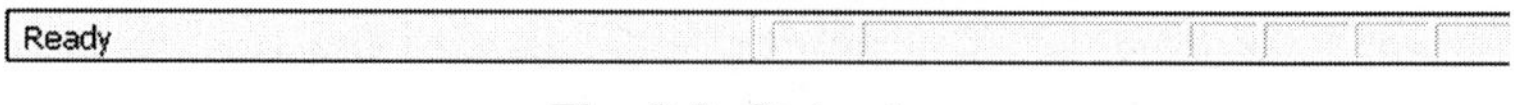

Fig. 6.8: Status bar

Notice the word “Ready” on the Status bar at the lower left side of the screen. The word “Ready” tells you that Excel is in the Ready mode and awaiting your next command. Other indicators appear on the Status bar in the lower right corner of the screen. Here are some examples:

The Down Arrow Key

You can use the down arrow key to move downward one cell at a time.

1. Press the down arrow key several times.
2. Note that the cursor moves downward one cell at a time.

The Up Arrow Key

You can use the Up Arrow key to move upward one cell at a time.

1. Press the up arrow key several times.
2. Note that the cursor moves upward one cell at a time.

The Tab Key

You can use the Tab key to move across the page to the right, one cell at a time.

1. Move to cell A1.
2. Press the Tab key several times.
3. Note that the cursor moves to the right one cell at a time.

The Right and Left Arrow Keys

You can use the right and left arrow keys to move right or left one cell at a time.

1. Press the right arrow key several times.
2. Note that the cursor moves to the right.
3. Press the left arrow key several times.
4. Note that the cursor moves to the left.

Moving Quickly Around the Worksheet

The following are shortcuts for moving quickly from one cell to a cell in a different part of the worksheet:

Go to — F5

The F5 function key is the "Go To" key. If you press the F5 key while in the Ready mode, you are prompted for the cell to which you wish to go. Enter the cell address and the cursor jumps to that cell.

1. Press F5. The Go To dialog box opens.
2. Type **J3**.
3. Press Enter. The cursor should move to cell J3.

Go to — Ctrl-G

You can also use Ctrl-G to go to a specific cell.

1. Hold down the Ctrl key while you press "g" (Ctrl-g). The Go To dialog box opens.
2. Type **C4**.
3. Press Enter. You should now be in cell C4.

Name Box

You can also use the Name box to go to a specific cell (**Fig. 6.9**).

1. Type **D10** in the Name box
2. Press Enter. You should now be in cell D10.

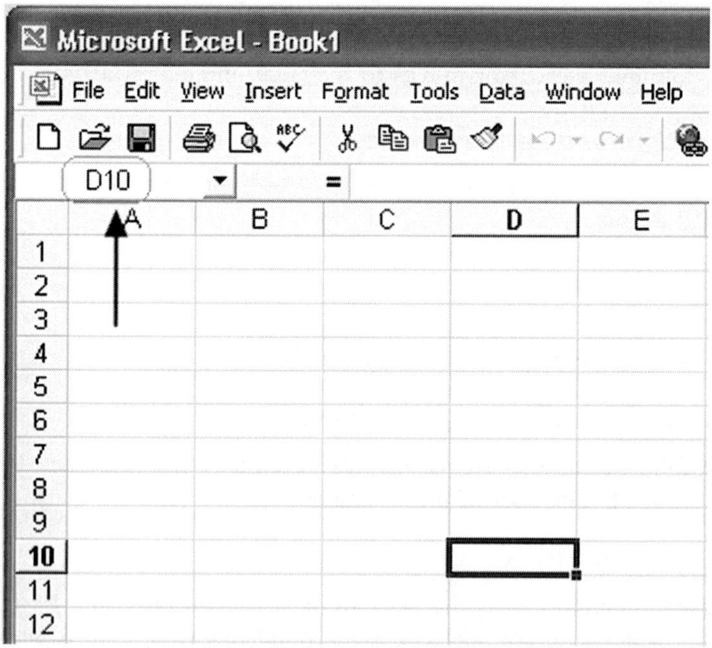

Fig. 6.9: Selecting a specific cell

Selecting Cells

If you wish to perform a function on a group of cells, you must first select those cells by highlighting them (**Fig. 6.10**). To highlight cells A1 to E1:

1. Place the cursor in cell A1.
2. Press the F8 key. This anchors the cursor.
3. Note that "EXT" appears on the Status bar in the lower right corner of the screen. You are in the Extend mode.
4. Click in cell E7. Cells A1 to E7 should now be highlighted.
5. Press Esc and click anywhere on the worksheet to clear the highlighting.

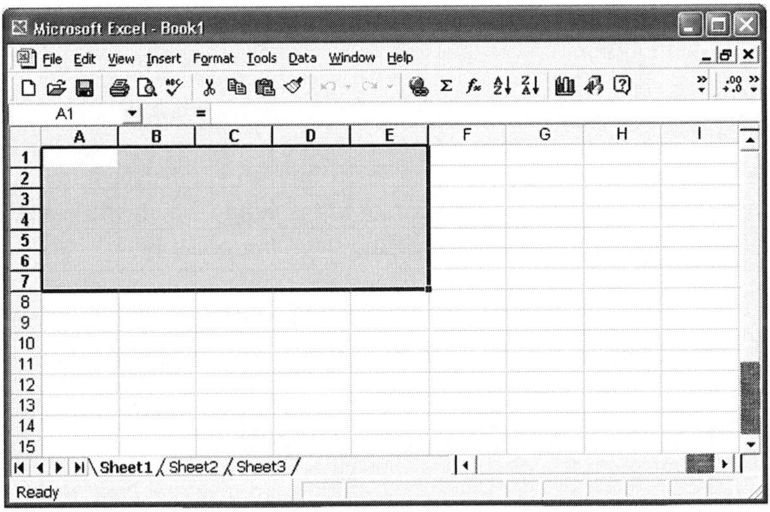

Fig. 6.10: Selecting a group of cells

Alternative Method: Selecting Cells by Dragging

You can also highlight an area by holding down the left mouse button and dragging the mouse over the area. In addition, you can select noncontiguous areas of the worksheet by doing the following:

1. Place the cursor in cell A1.
2. Hold down the Ctrl key. Do not release it until you are told. Holding down the Ctrl key enables you to select noncontiguous areas of the worksheet.

3. Press the left mouse button.
4. While holding down the left mouse button, use the mouse to move from cell A1 to E7.
5. Continue to hold down the Ctrl key, but release the left mouse button.
6. Using the mouse, place the cursor in cell G8.
7. Press the left mouse button.
8. While holding down the left mouse button, move to cell I17. Release the left mouse button.
9. Release the Ctrl key. Cells A1 to E7 and cells G8 to I17 are highlighted.
10. Press Esc and click anywhere on the worksheet to remove the highlighting.

ENTERING DATA

In this section, we are going to learn how to enter data into our worksheet. First, we place the cursor in the cell in which you would like to enter data. Then we type the data and press Enter.

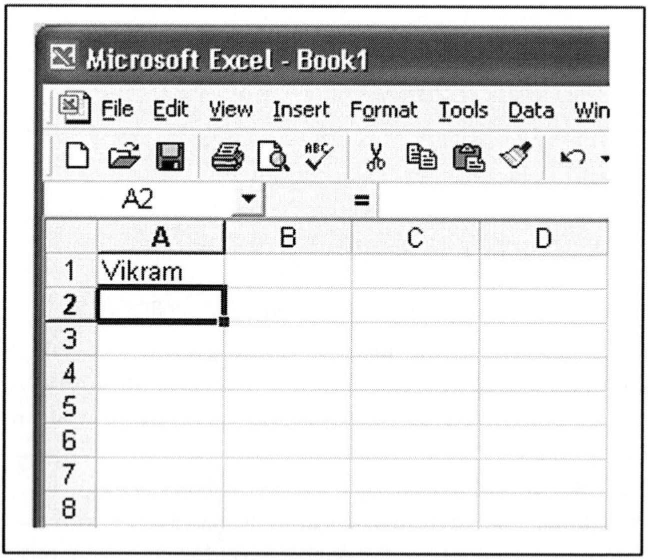

Fig. 6.11: Entering text in a cell

1. Place the cursor in cell A1.
2. Type **Vikram Duggal**.
3. The Backspace key erases one character at a time. Erase "Duggal" by pressing the backspace key until Duggal is erased.
4. Press Enter. The name "Vikram" should appear in cell A1 (**Fig. 6.11**).

Editing a Cell

After you enter data into a cell, you can edit it by pressing F2 while you are in the cell you wish to edit.

1. Move the cursor to cell A1.
2. Press F2.
3. Change "Vikram" to "Jones."
4. Use the backspace key to delete the name
5. Type **Jones**.
6. Press Enter (**Fig. 6.12**).

Alternate Method: Editing a Cell by Double-Clicking in the Cell

You can change "Jones" to "Johnson" as follows:

1. Move the cursor to cell A1.
2. Double-click in cell A1.

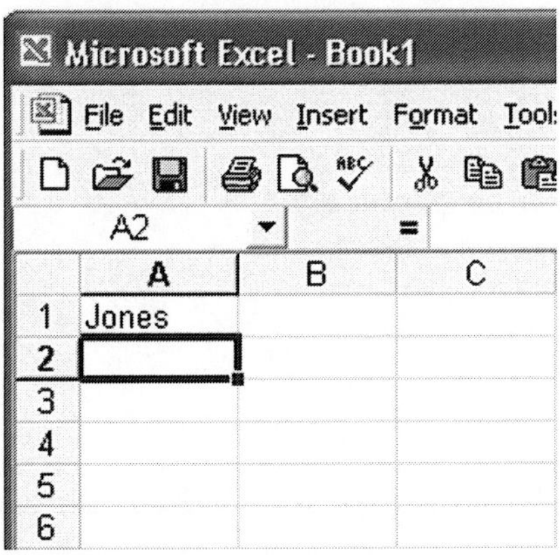

Fig. 6.12: Editing text in a cell

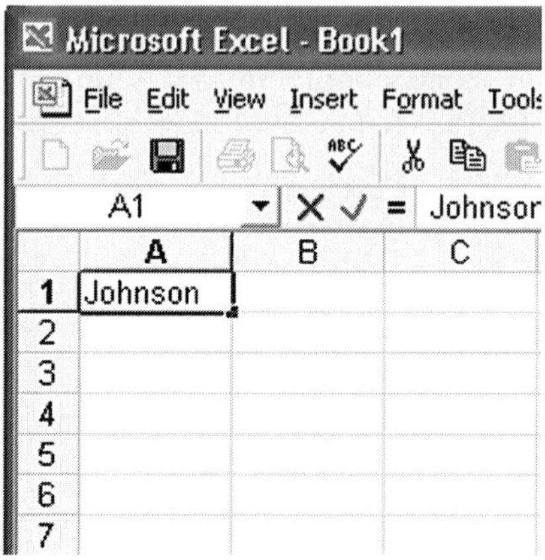

Fig. 6.13: Editing text in a cell

3. Press the End key. Your cursor is now at the end of your text.
4. Use the backspace to erase "n," "e," and "s".
5. Type **hnson**.
6. Press Enter (**Fig. 6.13**).

Wrapping Text

When you enter text that is too long to fit in a cell into a cell, it overlaps the next cell. If you do not want it to overlap the next cell you can wrap the text.

1. Move to cell A2.
2. Type **Text too long to fit**.
3. Press Enter.
4. Return to cell A2.
5. *Choose* Format > Cells *from the menu.*
6. Choose the Alignment tab.
7. Click Wrap Text.
8. Click OK. The text wraps.

Deleting a Cell Entry

To delete an entry in a cell or a group of cells, you place the cursor in the cell or highlight the group of cells and press Delete.

1. Place the cursor in cell A2.
2. Press the Delete key.

FORMATTING TEXT AND PERFORMING MATHEMATICAL CALCULATIONS

In this section, you are going to learn how to format text and perform basic mathematical calculations. To start, open a blank Microsoft Excel workbook.

Choosing a Default Font

Microsoft Excel enables you to choose a default font. The default font is the style of typeface that Excel will use unless you specify a different style. For the exercises in this lesson, you want your font to be set to Arial, Regular and Size 10. To set your font to Arial, Regular and Size 10:

1. *Choose* Format > Cells *from the menu.*
2. Choose the Font tab.
3. In the Font box, choose Arial.
4. In the Font Style box, choose Regular.
5. In the Size box, choose 10.
6. If there is no check mark in the Normal Font box, click to place a check mark there. Your selections are now the default.
7. Click OK.

Adjusting the Standard Column Width

When you open Microsoft Excel, the width of each cell is set to a default width. This width is called the standard column width. You need to change the standard column width to complete your exercises. To make the change, follow these steps:

1. *Choose* Format > Column > Standard Width *from the menu. The Standard Width dialog box opens.*
2. Type **25** in the Standard Column Width field. Click OK. The width of every cell on the worksheet should now be set to 25.
3. Move to cell A1.
4. Type **Cathy**.
5. Press Enter.

Cell Alignment

The name " Sharon" is aligned with the left side of the cell. You can change the cell alignment (**Fig. 6.14**).

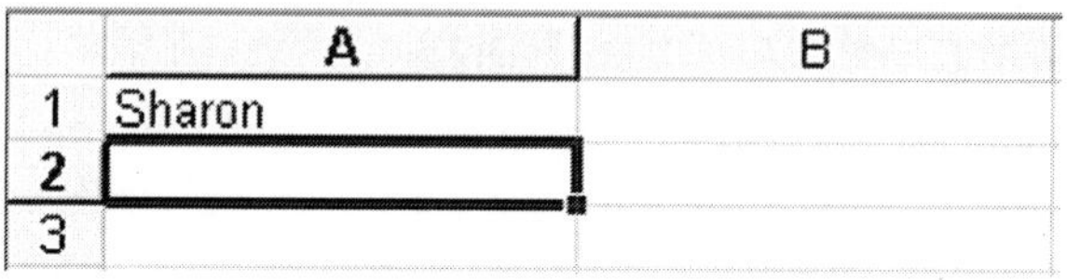

Fig. 6.14: Left-aligned text

Centering by Using the Menu

To center the name Cathy, follow these steps:

1. Move the cursor to cell A1.
2. *Choose* Format > Cells *from the menu. The Format Cells dialog box opens.*
3. Choose the Alignment tab.
4. Click to open the drop-down box associated with the Horizontal field. After the drop-down box is opened, click Center.
5. Click OK to close the dialog box. The name "Sharon" is centered (**Fig. 6.15**).

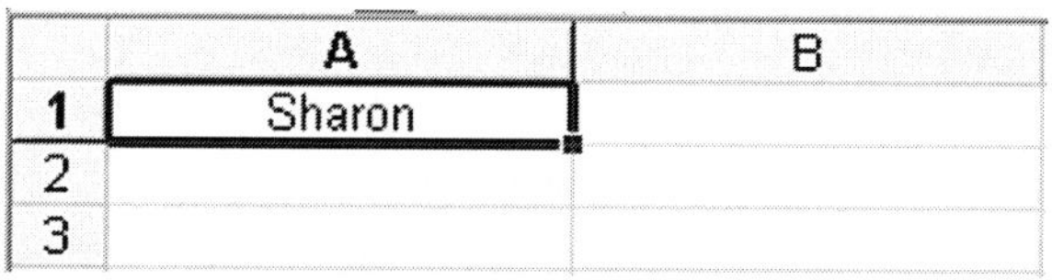

Fig. 6.15: Center-aligned text

Right-aligning by Using the Menu

To right-align the name "Sharon," follow these steps:

1. Move the cursor to cell A1.
2. *Choose* Format > Cells *from the menu. The Format Cells dialog box opens.*
3. Choose the Alignment tab.
4. Click to open the drop-down box associated with the Horizontal field. After the drop-down box opens, click Right (Indent).

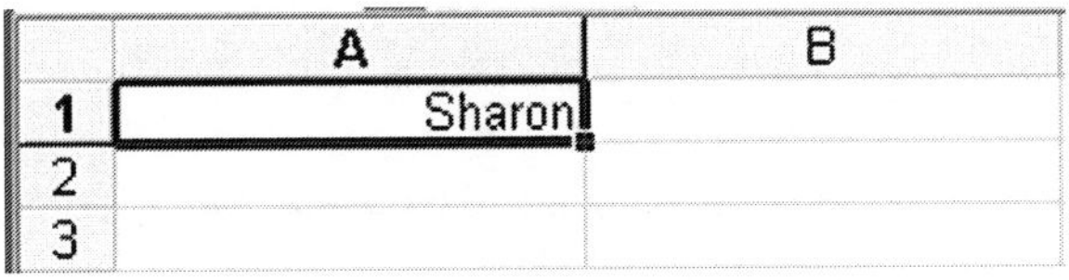

Fig. 6.16: Right aligned text

5. Click OK to close the dialog box. The name “Sharon” is right-aligned (**Fig. 6.16**).

Left-aligning by Using the Menu

To left-align the name “Sharon”, follow these steps:
1. Move the cursor to cell A1.
2. *Choose* Format > Cells *from the menu. The Format Cells dialog box opens.*
3. Choose the Alignment tab.
4. Click to open the drop-down box associated with the Horizontal field. After the drop-down box opens, click Left (Indent).
5. Click OK to close the dialog box. The name “ Sharon “ is left-aligned (**Fig. 6.17**).

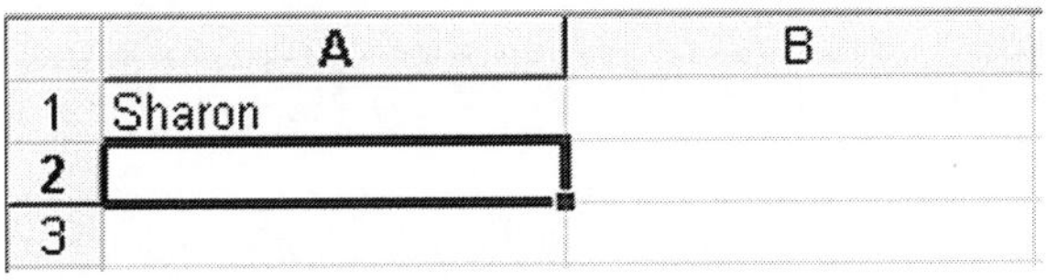

Fig. 6.17: The text is now left-aligned

Alternate Method: Alignment by Using the Formatting Toolbar

Using the Formatting toolbar, you can quickly perform tasks. You can use the Formatting toolbar to change alignment.

Centering by Using the Toolbar

To center the name “Cathy,” follow these steps:
1. Move the cursor to cell A1.
2. Click the Center icon, which is located on the Formatting toolbar (**Fig. 6.18**).

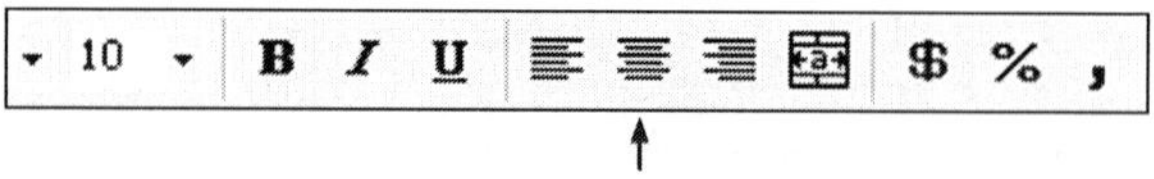

Fig. 6.18: The arrow points to the Align Center icon

Right-aligning by Using the Toolbar

You can right-align the name "Cathy" by following these steps:

1. Move the cursor to cell A1.
2. Click the Align Right icon, which is located on the Formatting toolbar (**Fig. 6.19**).

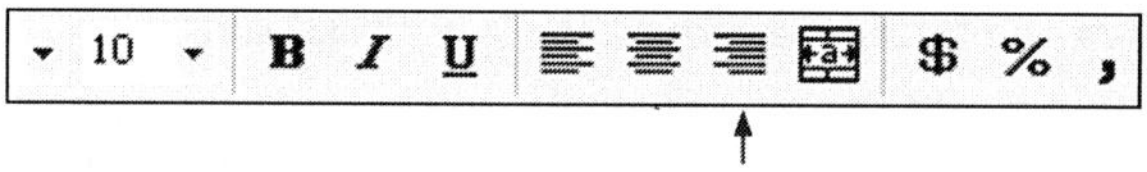

Fig. 6.19: The arrow points to the Align Right icon

Left-aligning by Using the Toolbar

You can left-align the name "Cathy" by following steps:

1. Move the cursor to cell A1.
2. Click the Align Left icon, which is located on the Formatting toolbar (**Fig. 6.20**).

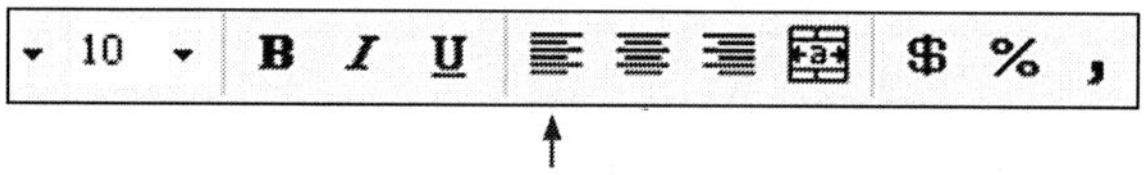

Fig. 6.20: The arrow points to the Align Left icon

Adding Bold, Underline and Italic

You can bold, underline or italicize text in Microsoft Excel. You can also combine these features. In other words, you can bold, underline and *italicize a single piece of text.*

There are three ways to bold, italicize and underline by using the menu, the icons and the shortcut keys.

Adding Bold by Using the Menu

1. Type **Bold** in cell A2.
2. Click the check mark located on the Formula bar. Clicking on the check mark is similar to pressing Enter (**Fig. 6.21**).

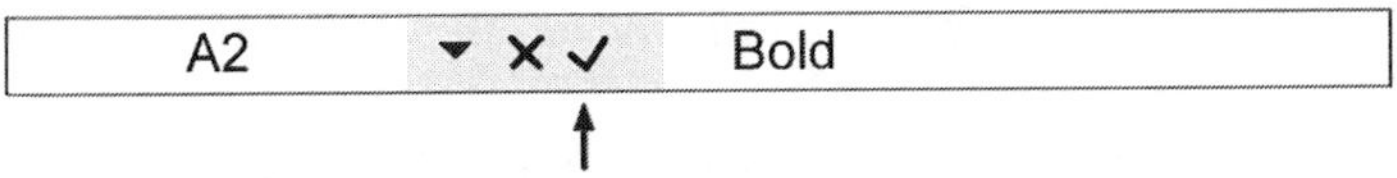

Fig. 6.21: Check mark is equivalent to hitting ENTER

3. *Choose* Format > Cells *from the menu. The Format Cells dialog box opens.*
4. Choose the Font tab.
5. Click Bold in the Font Style box.
6. Click OK. The word “Bold” should now be bolded.

Adding Italic by Using the Menu

1. Type **Italic** in cell B2.
2. Click the check mark located on the Formula bar. Clicking on the check mark is similar to pressing Enter.
3. *Choose* Format > Cells *from the menu. The Format Cells dialog box opens.*
4. Click Italic in the Font style box.
5. Click OK. The word “Italic” is italicized.

Adding Underline by Using the Menu

Microsoft Excel provides several types on underlines. The exercise that follows illustrates some of them:

Single Underline

1. Type **Underline** in cell C2.
2. Click the check mark located on the Formula bar. Clicking on the check mark is similar to pressing Enter.
3. *Choose* Format > Cells *from the menu. The Format Cells dialog box opens.*
4. Click to open the drop-down menu associated with the Underline box.
5. Click Single.
6. Click OK. The cell entry now has a single underline.

Double Underline

1. Type **Underline** in cell D2.
2. Click the check mark located on the Formula bar.

3. *Choose* Format > Cells *from the menu. The Format Cells dialog box opens.*
4. Click to open the drop-down menu associated with the Underline field.
5. Click Double.
6. Click OK. The cell entry now has a double underline.

Alternate Method: Adding Bold by Using the Icon

1. Type **Bold** in cell A3.
2. Click the check mark located on the Formula bar (**Fig. 6.22**).
3. Click the Bold icon, which is on the Formatting toolbar.
4. Click again on the Bold icon if you wish to remove the bolding.

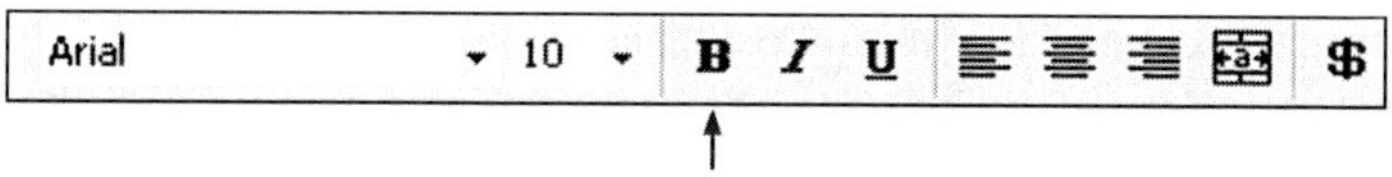

Fig. 6.22: The arrow points to the bold button

Alternate Method: Adding Italic by Using the Icon

1. Type **Italic** in cell B3.
2. Click the check mark located on the Formula bar (**Fig. 6.23**).
3. Click the Italic icon, which is on the Formatting toolbar.
4. Click again on the Italic icon if you wish to remove the italics.

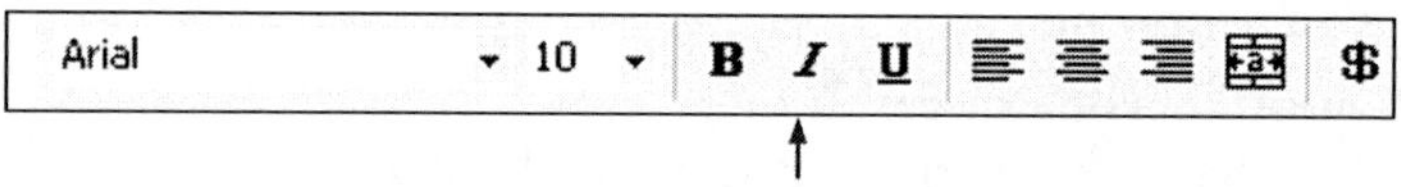

Fig. 6.23: The arrow points to the italics button

Alternate Method: Adding Underline by Using the Icon

1. Type **Underline** in cell C3.
2. Click the check mark located on the Formula bar (**Fig. 6.24**).
3. Click the Underline icon, which is on the Formatting toolbar.

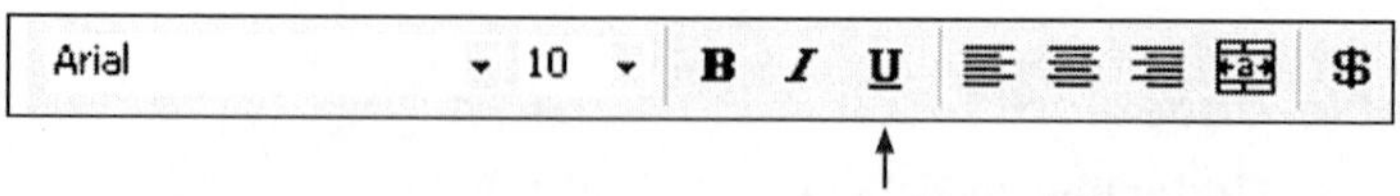

Fig. 6.24: The arrow points to the underline button

4. Click again on the Underline icon if you wish to remove the underline.

Changing the Font, Font Size and Font Color

You can change the font, font size and font color of the data you enter.

Changing the Font

1. Type **Times New Roman** in cell A5.
2. Click the check mark located on the Formula bar.
3. *Choose* Format > Cells *from the menu. The Format Cells dialog box opens.*
4. Choose the Font tab. All of the fonts listed in the Font box are available to you.

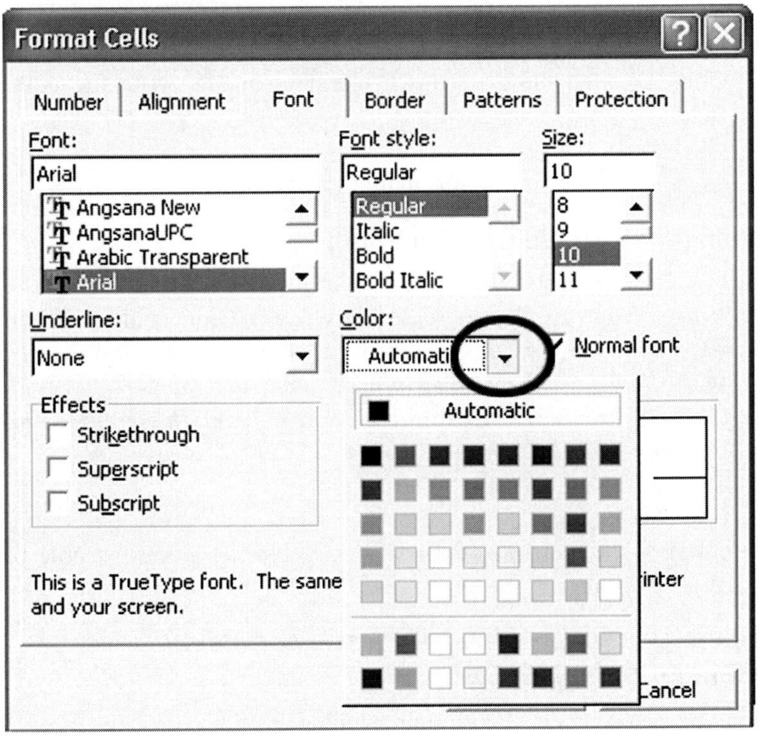

Fig. 6.25. Customizing font

5. Find and click Times New Roman in the Font box.
6. Click OK. The font changes from Arial to Times New Roman.

Changing the Font Size

1. Place the cursor in cell A5.
2. *Choose* Format > Cells *from the menu. The Format Cells dialog box opens.*
3. Choose the Font tab.
4. Click 16 in the Size box.
5. Click OK. The font size changes to 16.

Changing the Font Color

1. Place the cursor in cell A5.
2. *Choose* Format > Cells *from the menu. The Format Cells dialog box opens.*
3. Choose the Font tab (**Fig. 6.25**).
4. Click to open the drop-down menu associated with the color field.
5. Click Blue.
6. Click OK. The font color changes to blue.

Changing a Single Column Width

Earlier you increased the column width of every column on the worksheet. You can also increase individual column widths. If you increase the column width, you will be able to see the long text.

1. Make sure the cursor is anywhere under column A.
2. *Choose* Format > Column > Width *from the menu. The Column Width dialog box opens.*
3. Type **55** in the Column Width field.
4. Click OK.

Column A is set to a width of 55. You should now be able to see the whole text.

Alternate Method: Changing a Single Column Width by Dragging

You can also change the column width with the cursor.

1. Place the cursor on the line between the B and C column

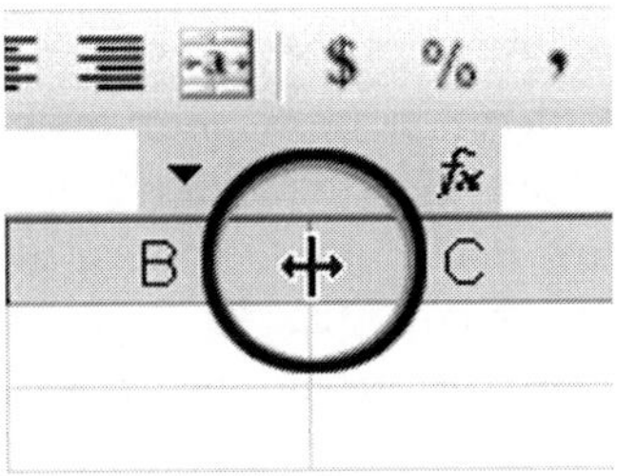

Fig. 6.26: Adjusting width of cells in a column

headings. The cursor should look like the one displayed here, with two arrows (**Fig. 6.26**).

2. Move your mouse to the right while holding down the left mouse button. The width indicator appears on the screen (**Fig. 6.27**).
3. Release the left mouse button when the width indicator shows approximately 40.

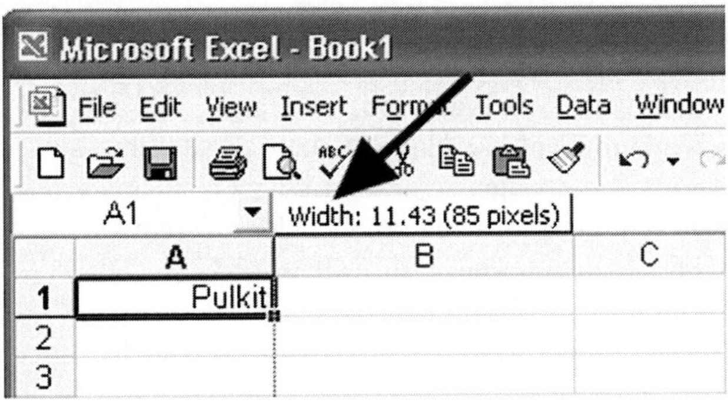

Fig. 6.27: The arrow points to width indicator

Moving to a New Worksheet

In Microsoft Excel, each workbook is made up of several worksheets. Before moving to the next topic, move to a new worksheet.

1. Click Sheet2 in the lower left corner of the screen (**Fig. 6.28**).

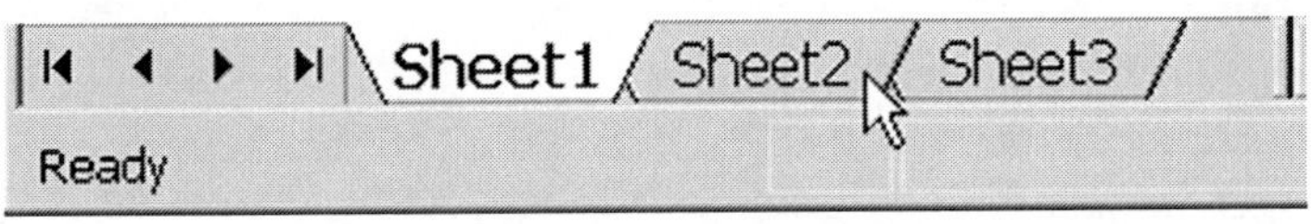

Fig. 6.28: Selecting sheets

Setting the Enter Key Direction

In Microsoft Excel, you can specify which direction the cursor moves when you press the Enter key. You can have the cursor move up, down, left, right or not at all. You will now make sure the cursor is set to move down when you press the Enter key.

1. *Choose* Tools > Options *from the menu. The Options dialog box opens.*
2. Choose the Edit tab.
3. Make sure there is a check mark in the "Move Selection after Enter" box.
4. If Down is not selected, click to open the Direction drop-down box. Click Down.
5. Click OK.

Making Numeric Entries

In Microsoft Excel, you can enter numbers and mathematical formulas into cells. When a number is entered into a cell, you can perform mathematical calculations such as addition, subtraction, multiplication and division. When entering a mathematical formula, precede the formula with an equal sign. Use the following to indicate the type of calculation you wish to perform:

+ Addition
– Subtraction
* Multiplication
/ Division
^ Exponential

Performing Mathematical Calculations

The following exercises demonstrate how to perform mathematical calculations:

Addition

1. Move your cursor to cell A1.
2. Type **1**.
3. Press Enter.
4. Type **1** in cell A2.

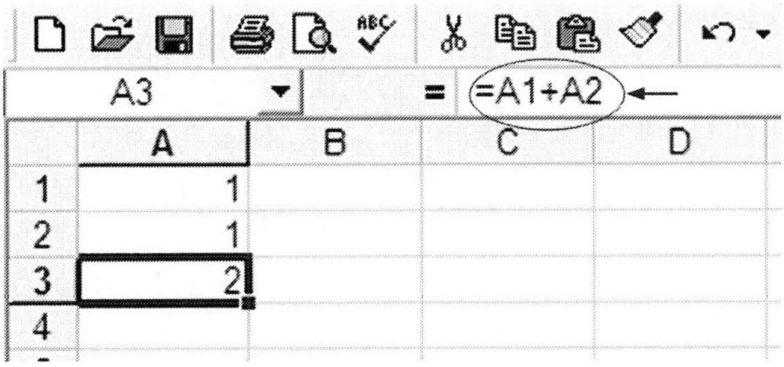

Fig. 6.29: Place the cursor in cell A3 and look at the Formula bar

5. Press Enter.
6. Type **=A1+A2** in cell A3.
7. Press Enter. Cell A1 has been added to cell A2 and the result is shown in cell A3 (**Fig. 6.29**).

Subtraction

1. Press F5. The Go To dialog box opens.
2. Type **B1** in the Reference field.
3. Press Enter. The cursor should move to cell B1.
4. Type **5** in cell B1.
5. Press Enter.
6. Type **3** in cell B2.
7. Press Enter.
8. Type =+**B1** – **B2** in cell B3.
9. Press Enter. Cell B1 has been subtracted from B2 and the result is shown in cell B3 (**Fig. 6.30**).

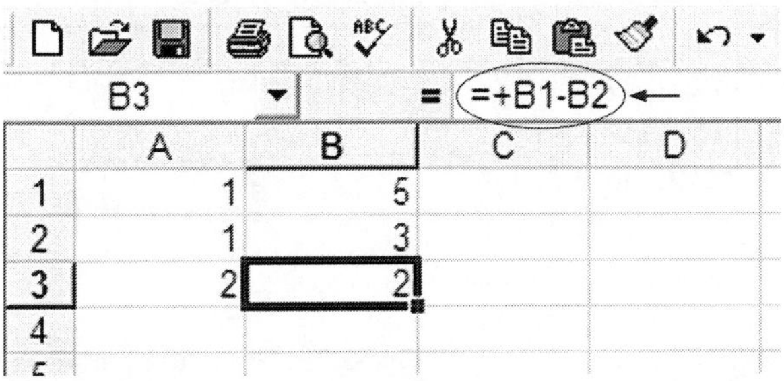

Fig. 6.30: Place the cursor in cell B3 and look at the Formula bar

Multiplication

1. Hold down the Ctrl key while you press "g" (Ctrl-g). The Go To dialog box opens.
2. Type **C1** in the Reference field.
3. Press Enter. You should now be in cell C1.
4. Type **2** in cell C1.
5. Press Enter.
6. Type **3** in cell C2.
7. Press Enter.
8. Type **=C1*C2** in cell C3.
9. Press Enter. Cell C1 is multiplied by cell C2 and the result is displayed in cell C3 (**Fig. 6.31**).

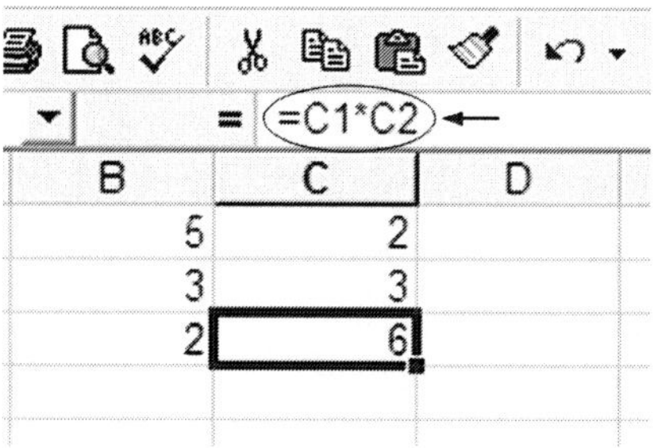

Fig. 6.31: Place the cursor in cell C3 and look at the Formula bar

Division

1. Press F5.
2. Type **D1** in the Reference field.
3. Press Enter. You should now be in cell D1.
4. Type **6** in cell D1.
5. Press Enter.
6. Type **3** in cell D2.
7. Press Enter.
8. Type =**D1/D2** in cell D3.
9. Press Enter. Cell D1 is divided by cell D2 and the result is displayed in cell D3 (**Fig. 6.32**).

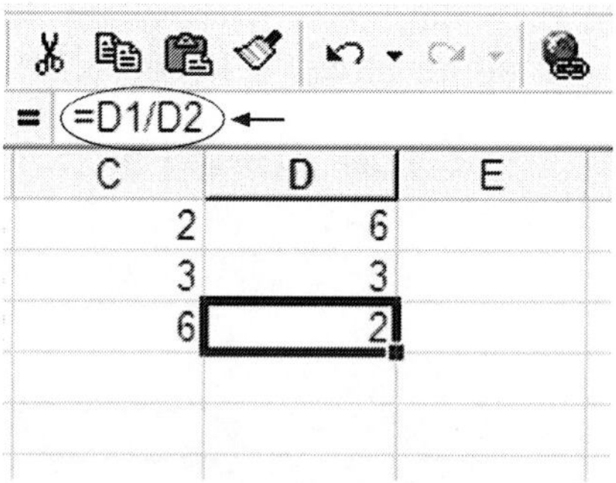

Fig. 6.32: Place the cursor in cell D3 and look at the Formula bar

The AutoSum Icon

The AutoSum icon on the Standard toolbar automatically adds a column of numbers. The following illustrates the SUM function:

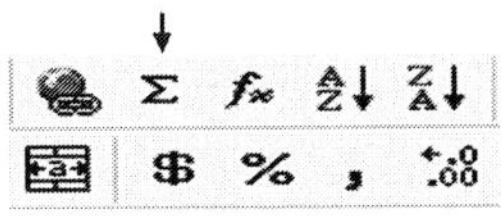

Fig. 6.33:
Autosum icon

1. Go to cell F1.
2. Type **3.** Press Enter.
3. Type **3**. Press Enter.
4. Type **3**. Press Enter.
5. Click the AutoSum button, which is located on the Standard toolbar (**Fig. 6.33**).
6. F1 to F3 should now be highlighted.
7. Press Enter. Cells F1 through F3 are added.

Automatic Calculation

If you have automatic calculation turned on, Microsoft Excel recalculates the worksheet as you change cell entries. You can check to make sure automatic calculation is turned on.

Setting Automatic Calculation

1. *Choose* Tools > Options *from the menu.*
2. Choose the Calculation tab.
3. Select Automatic if it is not already selected.
4. Click OK.

Trying Automatic Calculation

Make the changes outlined below and note how Microsoft Excel automatically recalculates.

1. Move to cell A1.
2. Type **2**. Press the Enter key. The results shown in cell A3 have changed. The number in cell A1 has been added to the number in cell A2 and the results display in cell A3.
3. Move to cell B1.

4. Type **6**.
5. Press the Enter key. The results shown in cell B3 have changed. The number in cell B1 has been subtracted from the number in cell B2 and the results display in cell B3.
6. Move to cell C1.
7. Type **4**. Press the Enter key. The results shown in cell C3 have changed. The number in cell C1 has been multiplied by the number in cell C2 and the results display in cell C3.
8. Move to cell D1.
9. Type ***12***. Press the Enter key. The results shown in cell D3 have changed. The number in cell D1 has been divided by the number in cell D2 and the results display in cell D3.

Deleting Columns

You can delete columns from your spreadsheet. To delete columns C and D (**Fig. 6.34**):

1. Click on column C and drag to column D.
2. *Choose* Edit > Delete *from the menu. Columns C and D are deleted.*
3. Click anywhere on the spreadsheet to remove your selection.

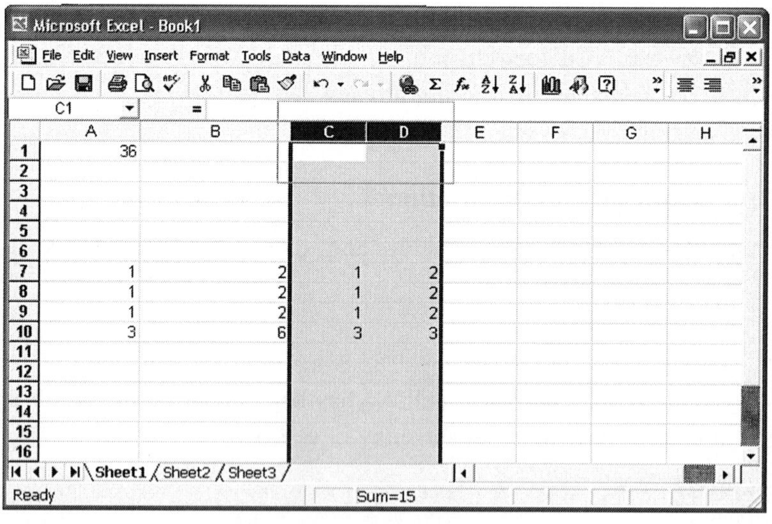

Fig. 6.34: Deleting columns

Deleting Rows

You can delete rows from your spreadsheet. To delete rows 1 through 4 (**Fig. 6.35**):

1. Click the row 1 and drag to row 4.
2. *Choose* Edit > Delete *from the menu. Rows 1 through 4 are deleted.*
3. Click anywhere on the spreadsheet to remove your selection.

Inserting Columns

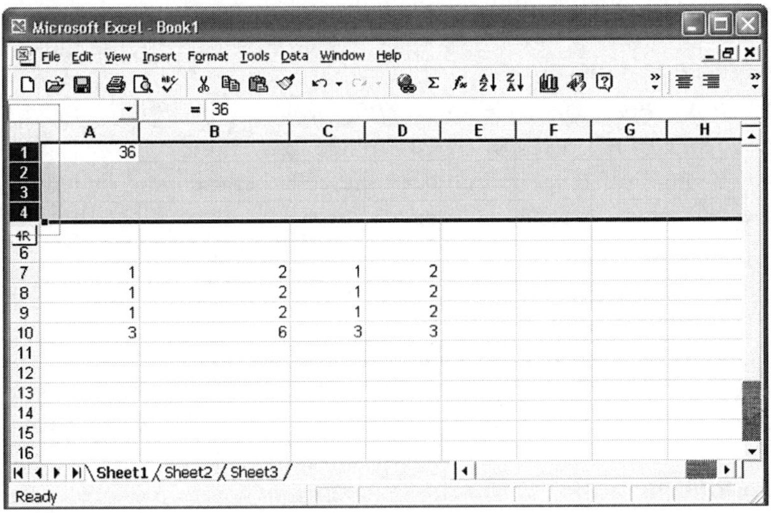

Fig. 6.35: Deleting rows

There will be times when you will need to insert a column or columns into your spreadsheet. To insert a column:

1. Click on A to select column A.
2. *Choose* Insert > Columns *from the menu. A column is inserted to the right of column A.*
3. Click anywhere on the spreadsheet to remove your selection.

Inserting Rows

You can also insert rows into your spreadsheet:

1. Click on 2 to select row 2.
2. *Choose* Insert > Rows *from the menu. A row is inserted above row 2.*
3. Click anywhere on the spreadsheet to remove your selection.

Numbers and Mathematical Calculations

Microsoft Excel has many functions that you can use. Functions allow you to quickly and easily find an average, the highest number, the lowest number, a count of the number of items in a list and make many other useful calculations.

Reference Operators

Reference operators refer to a cell or a group of cells. There are two types of reference operators, range *and* union.

A range reference refers to all the cells between and including the reference. A range reference consists of two cell addresses separated by a colon. The reference A1:A3 includes cells A1, A2 and A3. The reference A1:C3 includes A1, A2, A3, B1, B2, B3, C1, C2 and C3.

A union reference includes two or more references. A union reference consists of two or more cell addresses separated by a comma. The reference A7, B8, C9 refers to cells A7, B8 and C9.

Functions

Microsoft Excel has a set of prewritten formulas called functions. *Functions differ from regular formulas in that you supply the value but not the operators, such as +, –, * or /. For example, you can use the SUM function to add. When using a function, remember the following:*

- Use an equal sign to begin a formula.
- Specify the function name.
- Enclose arguments within parentheses.
- Use a comma to separate arguments.

Here is an example of a function:

=SUM(2,13,A1,B27)

In this function:

- The equal sign begins the function.
- SUM is the name of the function.
- 2, 13, A1 and B27 are the arguments.
- Parentheses enclose the arguments.
- A comma separates the arguments.

The SUM function adds the arguments together. In the exercises that follow, we will look at various functions.

Typing a Function

1. Open Microsoft Excel.
2. Type **12** in cell B1.
3. Press Enter.
4. Type **27** in cell B2.
5. Press Enter.
6. Type **24** in cell B3.
7. Press Enter.
8. Type **=SUM(B1:B3)** in cell A4.
9. Press Enter. Microsoft Excel sums cells B1 to B3.

Alternate Method: Entering a Function by Using the Menu

1. Type **150** in cell C1.
2. Press Enter.
3. Type **85** in cell C2.
4. Press Enter.
5. Type **65** in cell C3.
6. Press Enter. Your cursor should be in cell C4.
7. *Choose* Insert > Function *from the menu.*
8. Choose Maths and Trig in the menu Or Select Category box.
9. Click Sum in the Select A Function box.
10. Click OK. The Functions Arguments dialog box opens.
11. Type **C1:C3** in the Number1 field, if it does not automatically appear.
12. Click OK. Microsoft Excel sums cells C1 to C3.
13. Move to cell A4.

14. Type the word **Sum**.
15. Press Enter.

Calculating an Average

You can use the AVERAGE function to calculate the average of a series of numbers.

1. Move your cursor to cell A6.
2. Type **Average**.Press the right arrow key to move to cell B6.
3. Type = **AVERAGE(B1:B3)**.
4. Press Enter. The average of cells B1 to B3, which is 21, will appear.

Calculating an Average by Using the Sum Icon

In Microsoft Excel XP, you can use the Sum icon to calculate an average.

1. Move your cursor to cell C6.
2. Click the drop-down arrow next to the Sum icon.
3. Click Average.
4. Highlight C1 to C3.
5. Press Enter. The average of cells C1 to C3, which is 100, appears.

Calculating Minimum

You can use the MIN function to find the lowest number in a series of numbers.

1. Move your cursor to cell A7.
2. Type **Min**.
3. Press the right arrow key to move to cell B7.
4. Type = **MIN(B1:B3)**.
5. Press Enter. The lowest number in the series, which is 12 appears.

Calculating Maximum

You can use the MAX function to find the highest number in a series of numbers.

1. Move your cursor to cell A8.

2. Type **Max**.
3. Press the right arrow key to move to cell B8.
4. Type = **MAX(B1:B3)**.
5. Press Enter. The highest number in the series, which is 27, appears.

Note: You can also use the drop-down menu next to the Sum icon to calculate minimum and maximum.

Calculating Count

You can use the count function to count the number of items in a series.

1. Move your cursor to cell A9.
2. Type **Count**
3. Press the right arrow key to move to cell B9.
4. Click the down arrow next to the Sum icon.
5. Click Count.
6. Highlight B1 to B3.
7. Press Enter. The number of items in the series, which is 3 appears.

Filling Cells Automatically

You can use Microsoft Excel to fill cells automatically with a series. For example, you can have Excel automatically fill in times, the days of the week or months of the year, years and other types of series. Days of the week and months of the year fill in a similar fashion. The following demonstrates filling the days of the week:

1. Move to Sheet2.
2. Move to cell A1.
3. Type **Sun**.
4. Move to cell B1.
5. Type **Sunday**.
6. Highlight cells A1 to B1.
7. Bold cells A1 to B1.
8. Find the small black square in the lower right corner of the highlighted area. This is called the Fill Handle.

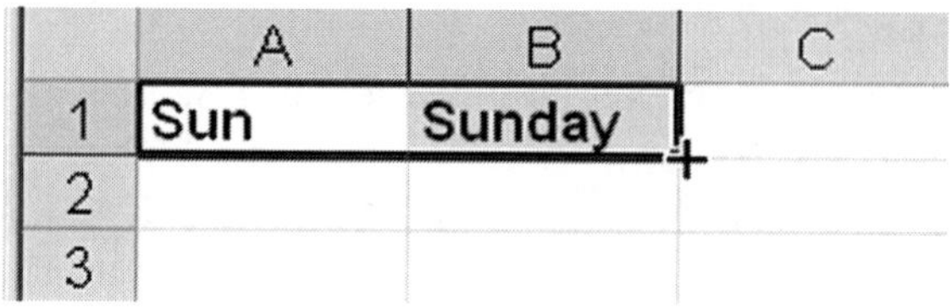

Fig. 6.36: Autofill cells

9. Grab the Fill Handle and drag with your mouse to fill cell A1 to B24. Note how the days of the week fill the cells in a series. Also, note that the Auto Fill Options icon appears (**Fig. 6.36**)
10. Click the Auto Fill Options icon.
11. Choose the Copy Cells radio button. The entry in cells A1 and B1 are copied to all the cells highlighted.
12. Click the Auto Fill Options icon again.
13. Choose the Fill Series radio button. The cells fill as a series from Sunday to Saturday again.
14. Click the Auto Fill Options icon again.
15. Choose the Fill without Formatting radio button. The cells fill as a series from Sunday to Saturday, but the entries are not bolded.
16. Click the Auto Fill Options icon again.
17. Choose the Fill Weekdays radio button. The cells fill as a series from Monday to Friday.

Some of the entries in column B are too long to fit in the column. You can quickly adjust the column width to fit the longest entry.

1. Move your cursor over the line that separates column B and C. The Width Indicator appears (**Fig. 6.37**).
2. Double-click. The column adjusts to fit the longest entry.

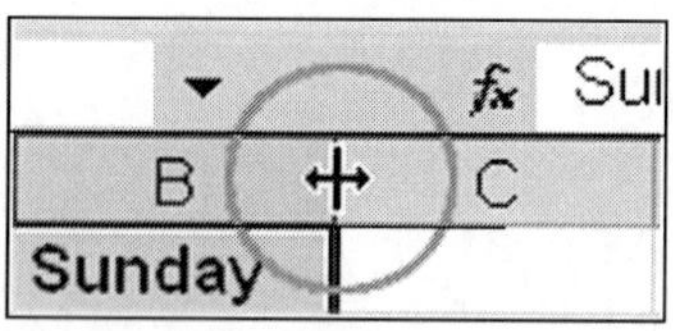

Fig. 6.37: Double click to adjust width automatically

The following demonstrates filling time:

1. Type **1:00** into cell C1.
2. Grab the Fill Handle and drag with your mouse to highlight cells A1 to A24. Note that each cell fills using military time.
3. Press Esc and then click anywhere on the worksheet to remove the highlighting.

To change the format of the time:

1. Select cells C1 to C24.
2. *Choose* Format > Cells *from the menu.*
3. Choose the Number tab.
4. In the Category box, choose Time.
5. In the Type box, choose 1:30 PM.
6. Click OK. The time is no longer in military time.

You can also fill numbers.

1. Type **1** in cell D1.
2. Grab the Fill Handle and drag with your mouse to highlight cells D1 to D24. The number 1 fills each cell.
3. Click the Auto Fill Options icon.
4. Choose the Fill Series radio button. The cells fill as a series starting with 1, 2, 3.

Here is another interesting fill feature:

1. Go to cell E1.
2. Type **Lesson 1**.
3. Grab the Fill Handle and drag with your mouse to highlight cells E1 to E24.
4. The cells fill in as a series: Lesson 1, Lesson 2, Lesson 3 and so on.

Printing

The simplest way to print is to click the Print icon located on the Standard toolbar. Dotted lines will appear on your screen after you click the print icon. The dotted lines indicate the right, left, top and bottom edges of your printed pages.

Creating Charts

Using Microsoft Excel, you can represent numbers in a chart. You can choose from a variety of chart types. And, as you change your data, your chart will automatically update. You can use Microsoft Excel's Chart Wizard to take you through the process step-by-step.

Creating a Column Chart

To create the column chart shown in **Figure 6.38** start by creating the spreadsheet below exactly as shown (**Fig. 6.39**).

After you have created the spreadsheet, you are ready to create your chart.

1. Highlight cells A3 to D6. You must highlight all the cells containing the data you want in your chart. You should also include the data labels.
2. *Choose* Insert > Chart *from the menu.*
3. Click Column to select the type of chart you want to create.
4. In the Chart Sub-type box, choose the Clustered Column icon to select the chart sub-type (**Fig. 6.40**).

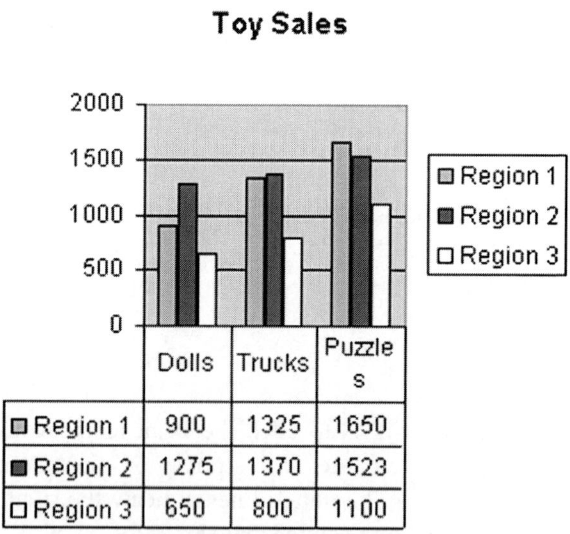

Fig. 6.38: A column chart

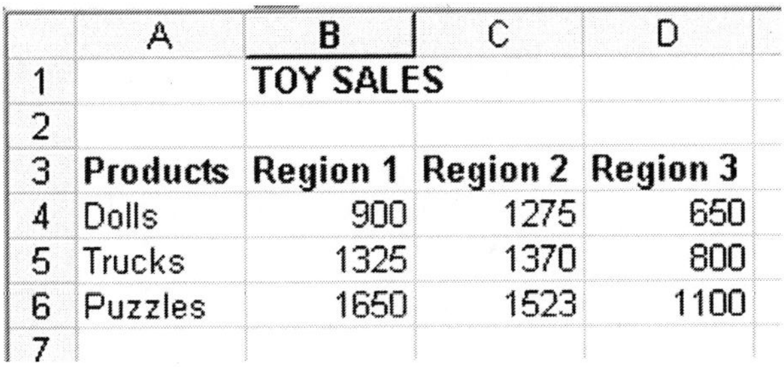

	A	B	C	D
1		TOY SALES		
2				
3	**Products**	**Region 1**	**Region 2**	**Region 3**
4	Dolls	900	1275	650
5	Trucks	1325	1370	800
6	Puzzles	1650	1523	1100
7				

Fig. 6.39: Entering data for a chart

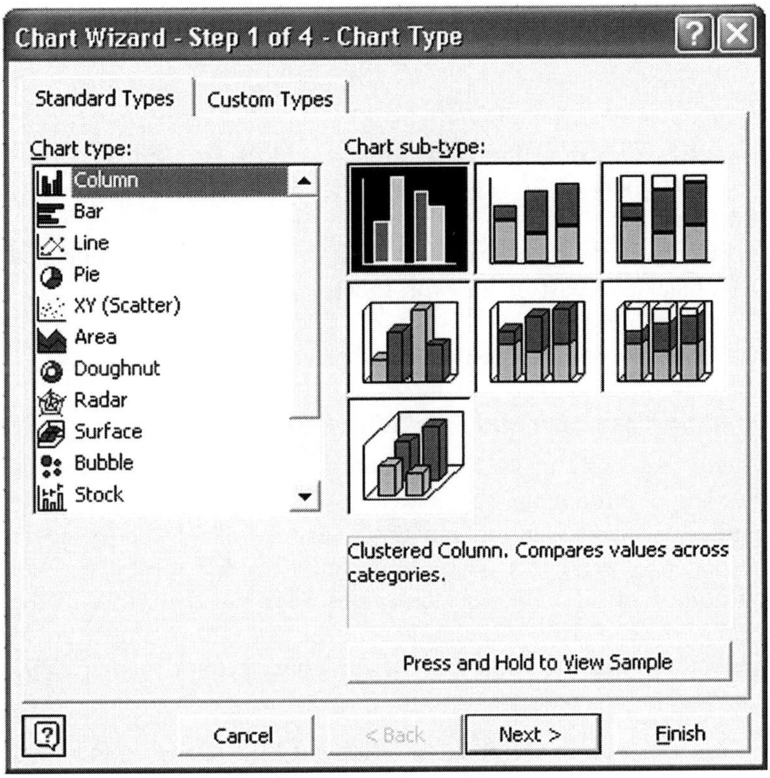

Fig. 6.40: Selecting chart type

5. Click Next.
6. To place the product names on the X-axis, select the Columns radio button.
7. Click Next.
8. Type Toy Sales in the Chart Title field. Toy Sales will appear as the title of your chart.
9. Type Products in the Category (X) Axis field. Products will appear as your x-axis title.
10. Type Units Sold in the Value (Y) Axis field. Units Sold will appear as your y-axis title.
11. Choose the Data Labels tab.
12. Select Value in the Labels Contain Frame to display the data labels as values.
13. Choose the Data Table tab.
14. Select Show Data Table. The data table will appear below your chart.
15. Click Next.
16. Choose As Object In Sheet1 to make your chart an embedded object and part of the worksheet.
17. Click Finish
18. Your chart will appear on the spreadsheet.

Changing the Size and Position of a Chart

When you select a chart, handles appear on the right and left sides, the top and bottom and the corners of the chart. You can drag the handles on the top and bottom of the chart to increase or decrease the height of the chart. You can drag the handles on the left and right sides of the chart to increase or decrease the width of the chart. You can drag the handles on the corners of the chart to increase or decrease the size of the chart proportionally (**Fig. 6.41**).

You can change the position of a chart by clicking on the chart and dragging.

1. Use the handles to adjust the size of your chart.
2. Click the chart and drag to position the chart under the data.

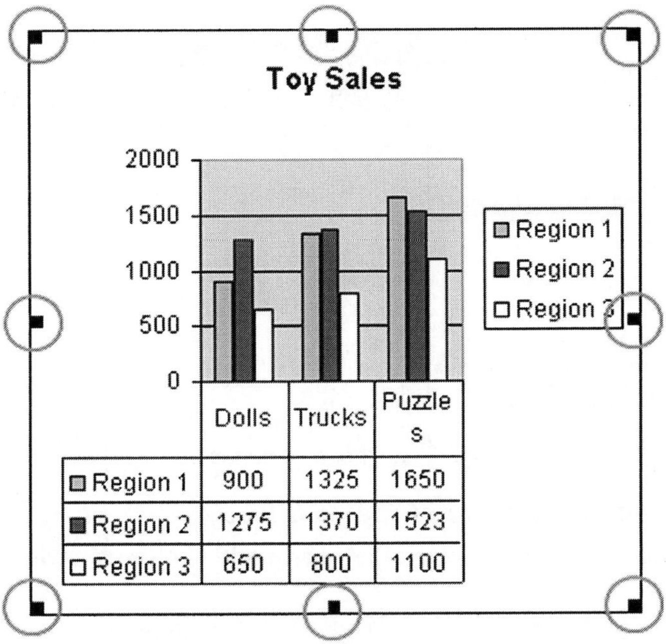

Fig. 6.41: Adjust size and position by using handles on the corners

Modify Your Chart

You can modify your chart by using the Chart toolbar. If the Chart toolbar is not already available, choose View > Toolbars > Chart from the menu (**Fig. 6.42**).

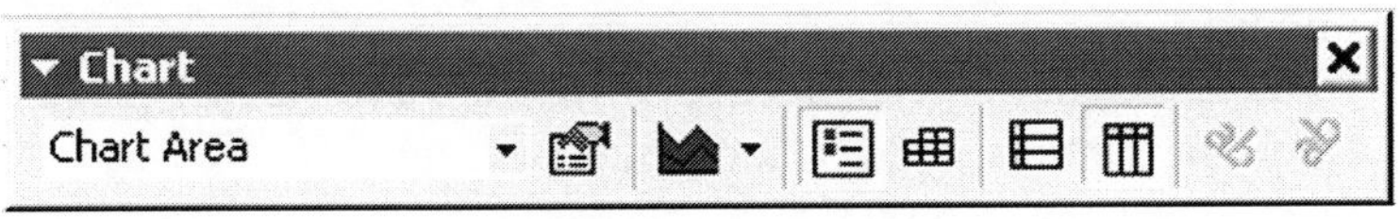

Fig. 6.42: Chart toolbar

To change the data area font size:

1. Click the down arrow on the Chart toolbar. A drop-down menu opens.
2. Choose Data Table from the drop-down menu (**Fig. 6.43**).
3. Click the Options icon. Choose the Font tab.
4. In the Size box, type 8.
5. Click OK. Your font size is now 8.

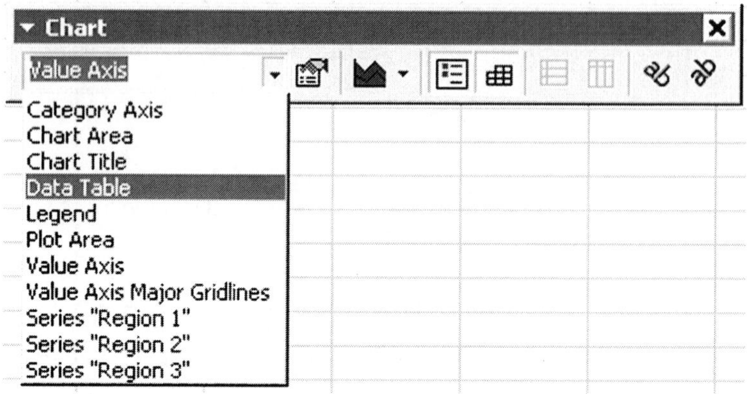

Fig. 6.43: Choose data table

To change the angle of the data labels:

1. Click the down arrow on the Chart toolbar. A drop-down menu opens.
2. Choose "Region 1" data labels from the drop-down menu.
3. Click the Angle Counter Clockwise icon  . The Region 1 data labels are angled counter-clockwise.
4. Repeat this process for Regions 2 and 3.

To change the font size of the Region data labels:

1. Click the down arrow on the Chart toolbar. A drop-down menu opens.
2. Choose "Region 1" Data Labels from the drop-down menu.
3. Click the Options icon. Choose the Font tab.
4. In the Size box, type 6.
5. Click OK. Your font size is now 6.
6. Repeat this process for Region 2 and 3.

You can also make changes by double-clicking on the item you want to change.

To change the chart scale:

1. Double-click on the scale. The Format Axis dialog box opens (**Fig. 6.44**).

2. Choose the Scale tab.
3. Type 400 in the Major Unit field.
4. Click OK. Your chart is now scaled in units of 400.

Saving Your File

To save your file:

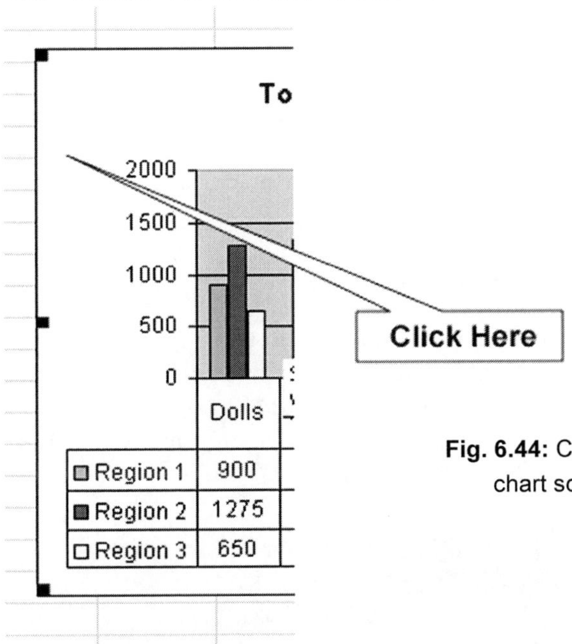

Fig. 6.44: Changing chart scale

1. *Choose* File>Save *from the menu.*
2. Go to the directory in which you want to save your file.
3. Type **arjun_table** in the File Name field.
4. Click Save.

Closing Microsoft Excel

Close Microsoft Excel by clicking on the cross on the upper right corner, or *Choose* File > **Exit** *from the menu.*

Seven

Introduction to Microsoft Powerpoint

INTRODUCTION

Microsoft PowerPoint is a powerful tool to create professional looking presentations and slide shows. PowerPoint allows you to construct presentations from scratch or by using the easy to use wizard.

Starting Microsoft PowerPoint

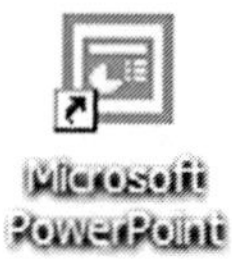

Fig. 7.1

There are two ways to do this

1. Double click on the Microsoft PowerPoint icon on the desktop **(Fig. 7.1)**
2. Click on Start —> Programs —> Microsoft PowerPoint (**Fig. 7.2**).

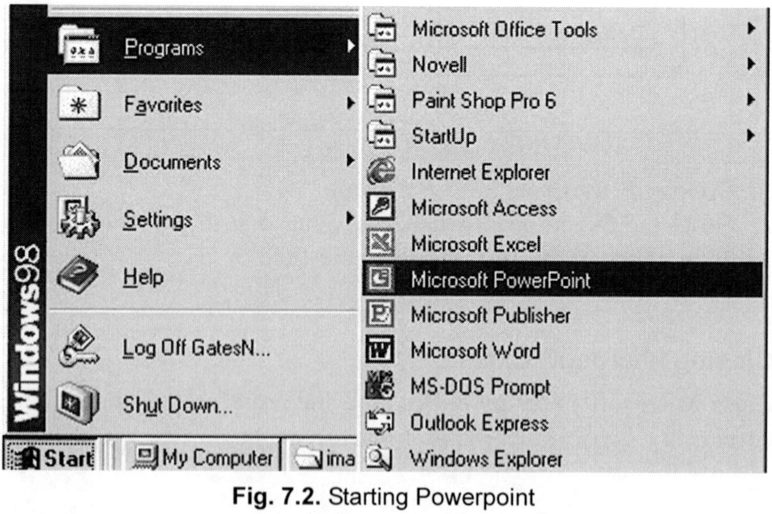

Fig. 7.2. Starting Powerpoint

The PowerPoint Screen

You use PowerPoint to create effective slide show presentations. The PowerPoint screen has many elements (Refer to **Fig. 7.3**).

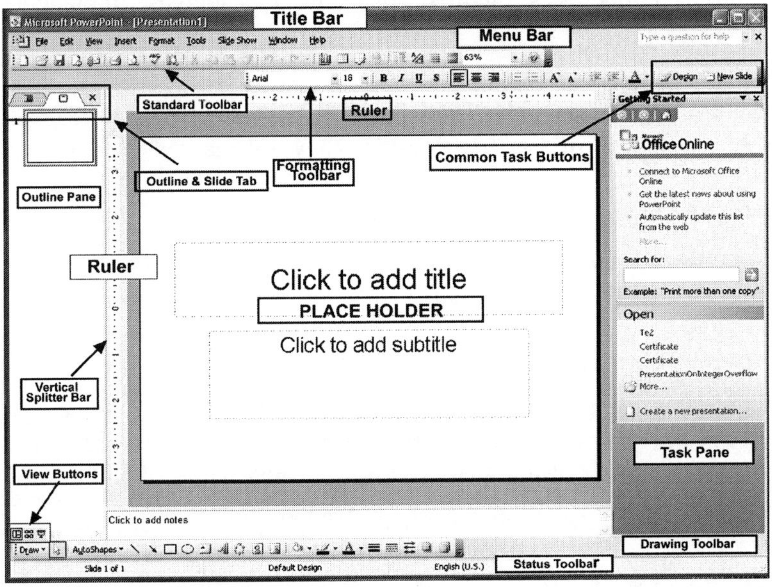

Fig. 7.3. The Powerpoint Screen

Title Bar

The Title bar generally appears at the top of the screen. The Title bar displays the title of the current presentation.

Menu Bar

The Menu bar displays the menu. You use the menu to give instructions to PowerPoint.

Standard and Formatting Toolbars

PowerPoint has several toolbars. Toolbars provide shortcuts to menu commands. The most commonly used toolbars are the Standard and Formatting toolbars. You use the Standard toolbar to do such things as open a file; save a file; print a file; check spelling; cut, copy and paste; undo and redo; or insert a chart or table. You use the Formatting toolbar to change the font, font size or font color; bold, underline or italicize text; left align, right align, center or justify; bullet or number lists; highlight; or decrease or increase the indent.

Rulers

Rulers are vertical and horizontal guides. You use them to determine where you want to place an object. They are marked in inches.

Placeholders

Placeholders hold the objects in your slide. You use placeholders to hold text, clip art and charts.

Status Bar

The Status bar generally appears at the bottom of the screen. The Status bar displays the number of the slide that is currently displayed, the total number of slides and the name of the design template in use or the name of the background.

Outline Tab

The Outline displays the text contained in your presentation.

Slides Tab

The Slides tab displays a thumbnail of all your slides. You click the thumbnail to view the slide in the Slide pane.

View Buttons

The View buttons appear near the bottom of the screen. You use the view buttons to change between Normal view, Slider Sorter view and the Slide Show.

Normal View

Normal view splits you screen into three major sections: the Outline and Slides tabs, the Slide pane and the Task pane. The Outline and Slides tabs are on the left side of your screen. They enable you to shift between two different ways of viewing your slides. The Slides tab shows thumbnails of your slides. The Outline tab shows the text on your slides. The Slide pane is located in the center of your screen. The Slide pane shows a large view of the slide on which you are currently working. The Task pane is located on the right side of your screen. The Tasks pane enables you to select the task you want to perform.

Slide Sorter View

Slide Sorter view enables you to view thumbnails of all your slides. In Slide Sorter view you can easily add, delete or change the order of your slides. When you are in Slide Sorter view, a special Formatting toolbar appears. It has options that allow you to make changes to your slides.

Slide Show

Use the Slide Show view when you want to view your slides, as they will look in your final presentation. When in Slide Show view:

- **Esc:** Returns you to the view you were using previously.
- **Left-clicking:** Moves you to the next slide or animation effect. When you reach the last slide, you automatically return to your last view.
- **Right-clicking:** Opens a pop-up menu. You can use this menu to navigate the slides, add speaker notes, select a pointer and mark your presentation.

Drawing Toolbar

The Drawing toolbar generally appears near the bottom of the screen. It contains tools for creating and editing graphics.

Common Tasks Buttons

Using the common tasks buttons, you can select the type of tasks you want to perform.

Task Pane

The Task pane enables you to select the specific task you want to perform.

Vertical Splitter Bar

You can click and drag the vertical splitter bar to change the size of your panes.

Minimize Button

You use the Minimize button to remove a window from view. While a window is minimized, its title appears on the taskbar.

Maximize/Restore Button

You use the Maximize button to cause a window to fill the screen. After you maximize a window, if you click the Restore button, the window returns to its former size.

Close Button

You use the Close button to exit the window and close the program.

PowerPoint Overview

When you start PowerPoint, PowerPoint displays the Title Slide in the Slide pane. You can type the title of your presentation and a subtitle on this side. To enter text on the Title Slide:

- Click and type the title of your presentation in the "Click to add title" area.
- Click and type a subtitle in the "Click to add subtitle" area.

If you do not wish to use the Title Slide, choose Edit > Delete *slide from the menu to delete it.*

Create New Slides

After completing your title slide, you can create additional slides. To create a new slide:

1. Do one of the following:

- *Choose* Insert > New Slide *from the menu.*
- Click the New Slide button
- Press Ctrl-M.

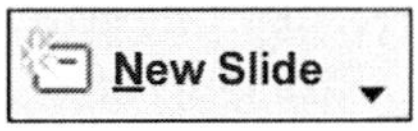

The Apply Slide Layout pane will appear on the right side of the screen. The Apply Slide Layout pane provides you with slide templates you can use when creating your PowerPoint presentation. There are four types of Text Layout templates.

- **Title Slide** – The Title Slide contains two text placeholders that you can use to display a title and a subtitle of your presentation.
- **Title Only** – The Title Only slide contains a single placeholder. You can use it to display a title.
- **Title and Text** – The Title and Text template provides a placeholder for a title and a placeholder for text.
- **Title and 2 Column Text** – The Title and Text template provides a placeholder for a title and two placeholders for text.

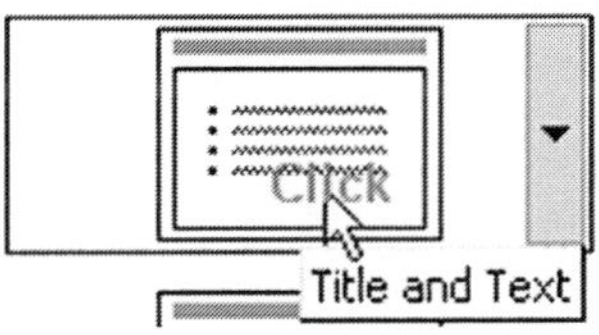

Fig. 7.4

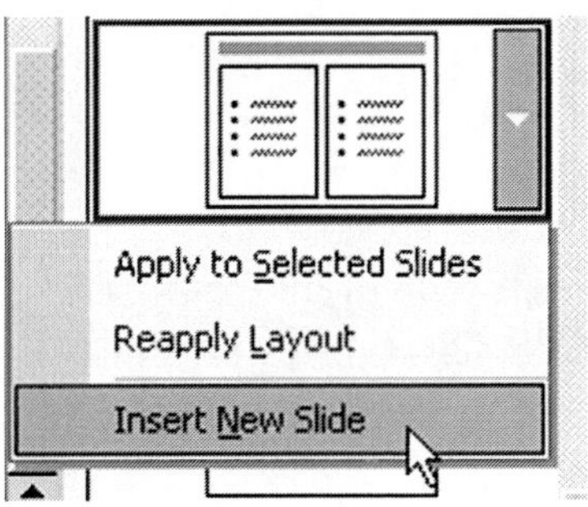

Fig. 7.5

2. To select a layout, click the layout you want in the Apply Slide Layout pane. The layout will then appear in the Slide pane. (Refer to **Fig. 7.4**)
3. To add text, click inside the placeholder and type.
4. To add an additional slide to your presentation do one of the following:
   - *Right-click on the slide layout. A menu will appear. Choose* Insert New Slide.
   - *Click the down arrow next to the slide layout.*

A menu will appear). Choose Insert New Slide *(Refer to* ***Fig.*** *7.5)*

Change Your Slides

After creating a slide, if you want to add text:

1. Place the cursor at the point at which you would like to add text.
2. Type the information you want to add.

If you would like to change text:

1. Highlight the text you want to change.
2. Type the new text.

You can use the backspace key to delete text. You can also delete text by highlighting the text and pressing the Delete key.

Apply a Design Template

Design templates provide attractive backgrounds for your PowerPoint slides. To apply a design template:

1. Do one of the following:
   - *Choose* Format > Slide Design *from the menu.*
   - Click the Slide Design icon 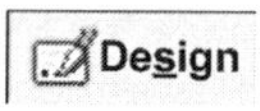

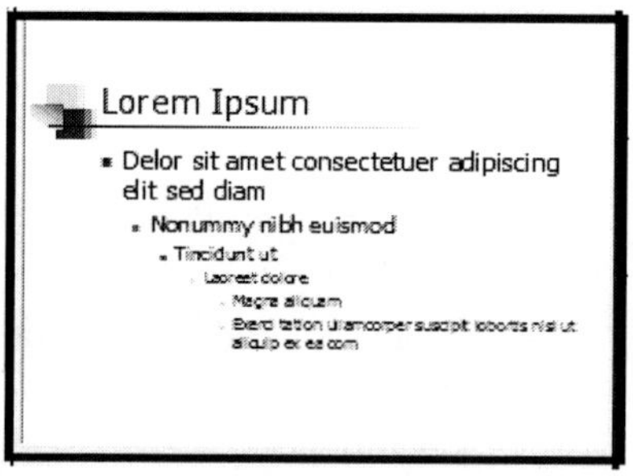

Fig. 7.6

Design templates will appear on the right side of the screen.

2. To apply a design template to all of the slides in your presentation do one of the following:
   - Click on the design template.
   - *Right-click on the template. A menu will appear. Choose* Apply to All Slides.

- *Click on the down arrow next to the template. A menu will appear. Choose* Apply to All Slides *(Refer to **Fig. 7.6**).*

Correct Spelling

Using the PowerPoint spell checker, you can check the spelling in you PowerPoint documents.

1. To start spell check, do one of the following:
    - *Choose* Tools > Spelling *from the menu.*
    - Press F7.
    - Click the Spell Check icon.

    If there are possible spelling errors, the Spelling dialog box will open.

    - **Do not change spelling:** Click Ignore.
    - **Correct spelling:**
        1. Click the correct spelling in the Suggestions box.
        2. Click Change.
    - **Add to dictionary:** Click Add.
    - **Word is correct. Do not change document:** Click Ignore All.
    - **Word is incorrect. Change entire document:** Click Change All.

Sorter View

After you have created your PowerPoint slides, you can move, cut, copy, paste, duplicate, navigate and view them in Sorter view refer to **Fig. 7.7**. To view the slides in Sorter view, do one of the following:

- *Choose* View > Slide *Sorter from the menu.*
- Click the Slide Sorter View icon.

Run Your PowerPoint Slide Show

Once you have created your slides, you can run your Slide Show.

1. Do any one of the following:
    - Press F5.
    - *Choose* Slide Show > View Show *from the menu.*
    - Click the Slide Show icon, which is located in the bottom left corner of your screen.

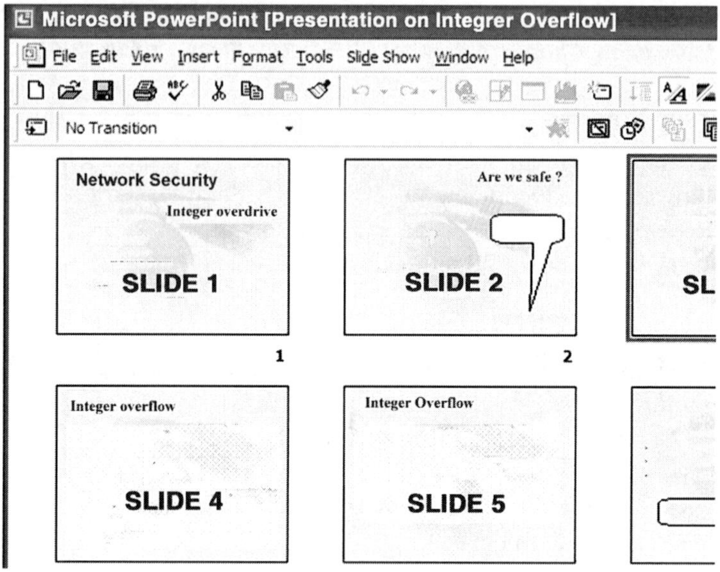

Fig. 7.7

Your slideshow will appear on your screen.

Table 7.1: Navigating the slideshow

Task	Procedure
Go to the next slide	Do one of the following: • Press the Right Arrow key • Press the Enter key • Press the Page Down key • Left-click
Go to the previous slide	Do one of the following: • Press the Left Arrow key • Press the Backspace key • Press the Page Up key

Print Your Slides

PowerPoint provides you with many printing options. You can print a large view of your slides or you can print your slides as handouts with 1, 2, 3, 4, 6 or 9 slides per page. You can also print your Notes pages or the Outline view of your slides.

Table 7.2: Slide sorter view

Task	**Procedure**
Move to first slide	Ctrl-Home
Move to last slide	Ctrl-End
Move to next slide	Right arrow
Move to previous slide	Left arrow
Select a slide	Single-click
Open slide in Normal view	Double-click slide
Select slides	Select a single slide: 1. Click the slide you want to select. Select multiple slides: 1. Hold down Ctrl key 2. Click the slides you want to select
Delete a slide	1. Select the slide or slides you want to delete 2. Press the Delete key Or 1. Select the slide or slides you want to delete 2. *Choose* Edit > Delete Slide *from the menu*
Copy a slide	1. Select the slide 2. *Choose* Edit > Copy *from the menu* Or 1. Select the slide 2. Click the copy icon Or 1. Select the slide 2. Press Ctrl-C
Paste a slide	1. Select the slide after which you want the new slide or slides to appear 2. *Choose* Edit > Paste *from the menu* Or 1. Select the slide after which you want the new slide or slides to appear 2. Click the paste icon Or 1. Select the slide after which you want the new slide or slides to appear 2. Press Ctrl-V
Cut a slide	1. Select the slide or slides you want to cut 2. *Choose* Edit > Cut *from the menu* Or 1. Select the slide or slides you want to cut 2. Click the Cut icon Or 1. Select the slide or slides you want to cut 2. Press Ctrl-X
Move a slide	1. Select the slide or slides you want to move. 2. Drag to the new location
Duplicate a slide	1. Select the slide or slides you want to duplicate 2. *Choose* Edit > Duplicate *from the menu* Or 1. Select the slide or slides you want to duplicate 2. Press Ctrl-D

To print:

1. *Choose* File >Print Preview *from the menu. The Print Preview area will open.*
2. Click the down arrow next to the Print What field.
3. Select what you would like to print.
4. Click the Print icon. The Print dialog box will open.
5. Select whether you want your slides to print in color, grayscale or black and white. If you are using a black and white printer, choose black and white. You will use less ink or toner.
6. Check whether you want your slides to print vertically or horizontally.

Creating Your First PowerPoint Presentation

The following exercise steps you through creating your first PowerPoint presentation:

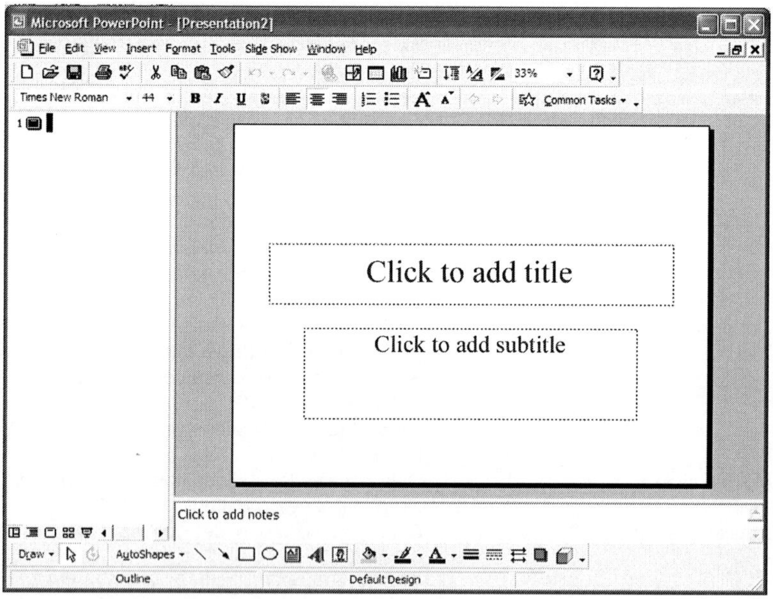

Fig. 7.8

Create a Title Slide

1. Open PowerPoint.
2. *Choose* Blank Presentation *on the Task pane. You will be presented with a Title slide (Refer to* ***Fig.*** *7.8).*
3. Enter the information shown here. Type College Scholarships and Financial Aid in the Click to Add Title box. Type Paying for College in the Click to Add Subtitle box (Refer to **Fig. 7.9**).

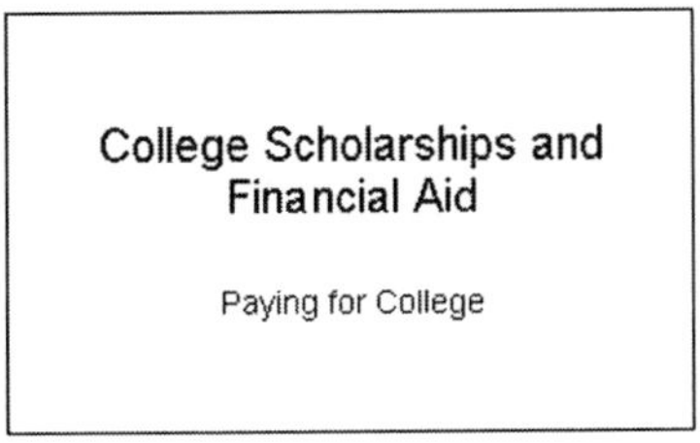

Fig. 7.9

Insert a New Slide

1. Click the New Slide icon 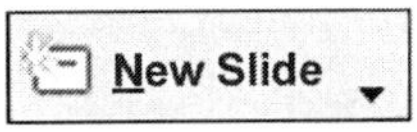

2. Click the Title and Text icon (Refer to **Fig. 7.10**).

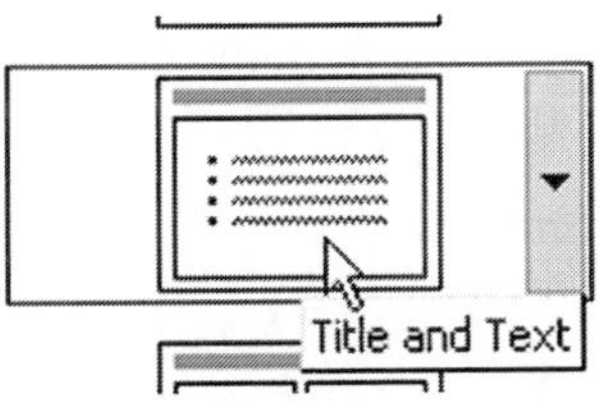

Fig. 7.10

3. Enter the information shown here. Type Here is what to do: in the Click to Add Title area. Type the bulleted text in the Click to Add Text area (Refer to **Fig. 7.11**).

Create a Hierarchy

1. Insert a new slide. Right-click the Title and Text icon. A context menu will appear. Choose *Insert New Slide* from the context menu.
2. Enter the information shown here (Refer to **Fig. 7.12**). Click the Increase Indent icon 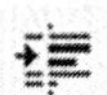 to indent the bullets for 'Stafford Loans' and 'PLUS Loans.' If you ever need to decrease an indent, use the decrease indent icon 

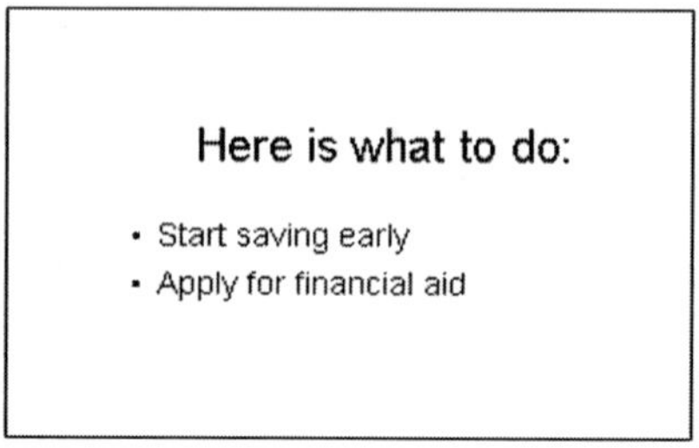
Here is what to do:
• Start saving early
• Apply for financial aid

Fig. 7.11

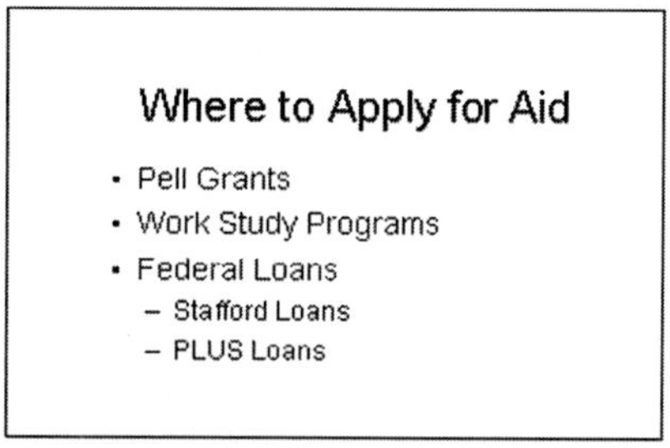

Fig. 7.12

Use Two-column Text

1. *Right-click the Title and 2 Column Text icon. A context menu will appear. Choose* Insert New Slide.
2. Enter the information shown here. Type the information in the appropriate column (Refer to **Fig. 7.13**).

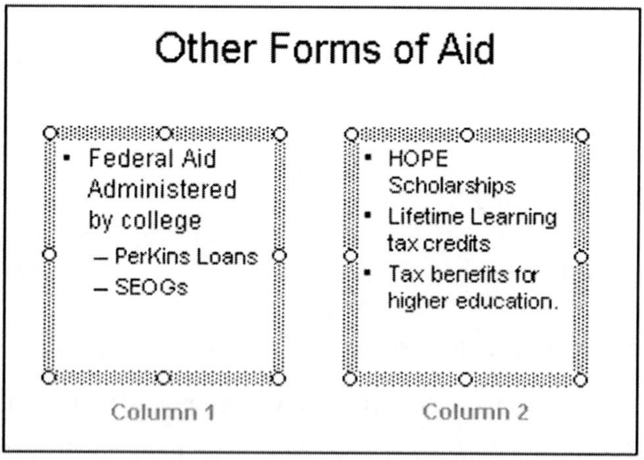

Fig. 7.13

Apply a Design Template

1. Click the design icon 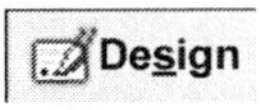 . Design templates will appear on the left side of the screen.
2. Scroll down to view the design templates.
3. *Right-click the design template you want to apply. A context menu will appear. Choose* Apply to All Slides. *We used the Lock and Key design template (Refer to* **Fig.** *7.14).*

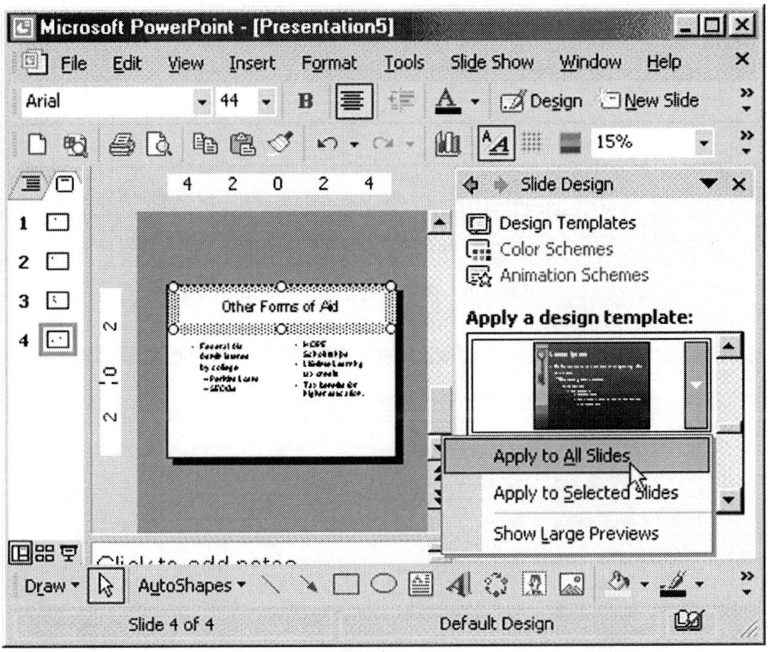

Fig. 7.14

Outline and Slides Tab

1. Use the Slides tab to view thumbnails of your slide (Refer to **Fig. 7.15**).
2. Click the Outline tab to view the text of your presentation as an outline (Refer to **Fig. 7.16**).

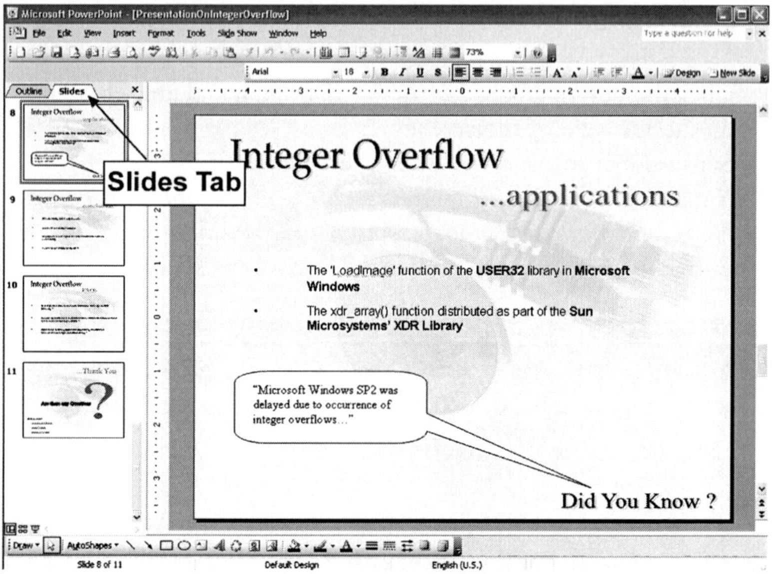

Fig. 7.15

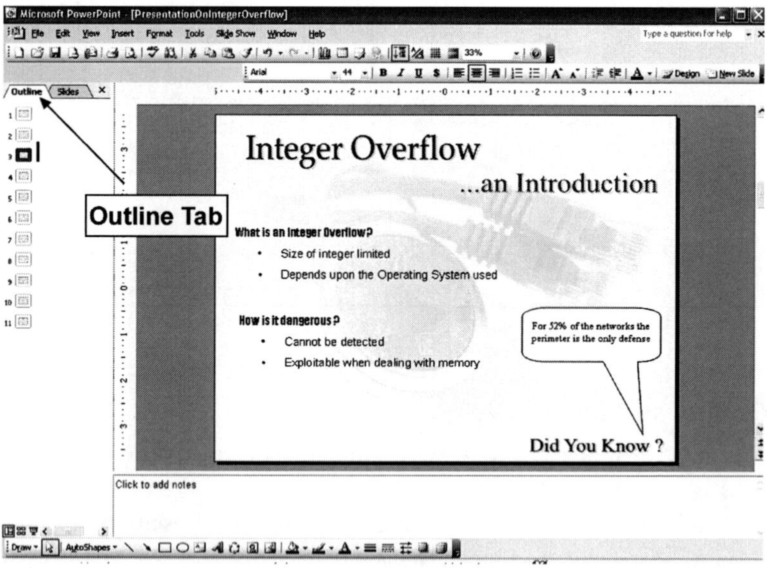

Fig. 7.16

Slide Sorter View

1. *Choose* View > Slide Sorter *from the menu to move to Slide Sorter view (Refer to* ***Fig. 7.17****).*
2. Double-click a slide to return to Normal view.

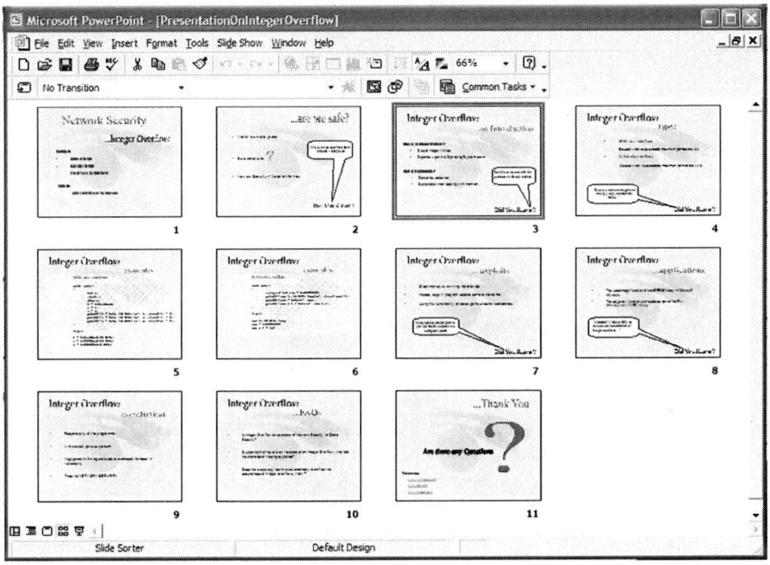

Fig. 7.17

Run Your Slide Show

1. Press F5 to run the Slide Show.
2. Use the arrow keys on your keyboard to move forward and backward through your slides.
3. Use the Esc key to return to Normal view.

Print Your Outline

1. *Choose* File > Print Preview *from the menu.*
2. Click the down arrow next to the Print What icon (Refer to **Fig. 7.18**).
3. Select Outline view (Refer to **Fig. 7.19**).
4. Click the Print icon.
5. Click Close.

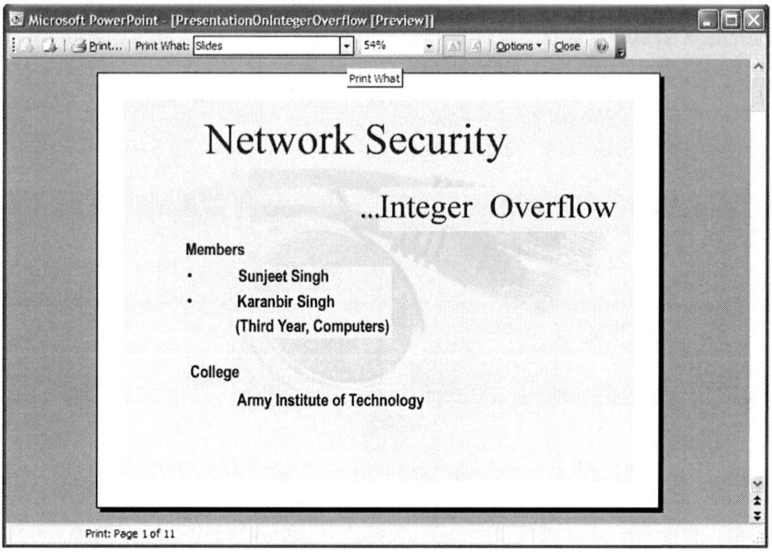

Fig. 7.18

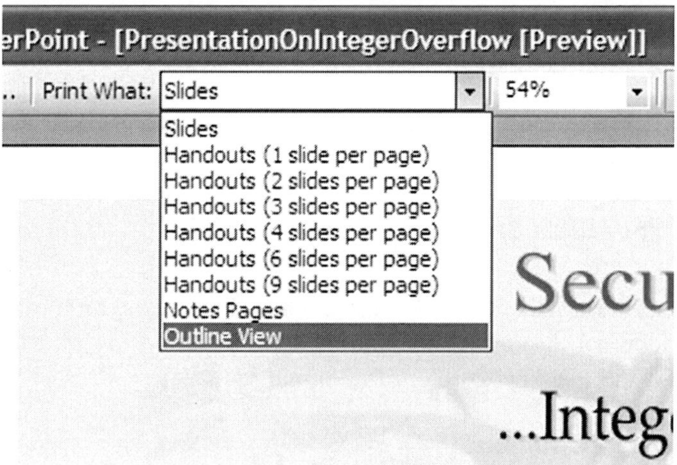

Fig. 7.19

Print Your Slides

1. *Choose* File > Print Preview *from the menu.*
2. Click the down arrow next to the Print What icon.
3. Select the slides you want to print.

4. Click the down arrow next to Options. A menu will appear.
5. *Choose* Color/Grayscale > Pure Black and White.
6. Click the Print icon.
7. Click Close.

Print Your Slides as a Handout

1. *Choose* File > Print Preview *from the menu.*
2. Click the down-arrow next to the Print What icon.
3. Select Handouts (2 slides per page).
4. Click the Print icon.
5. Click Close.

Eight

Introduction to Internet

INTRODUCTION TO INTERNET

Sometime in the mid 1960s, during the Cold War, it became apparent that there was a need for a bombproof communications system. A concept was devised to link computers together throughout the USA. With such a system in place large sections of the country could be nuked and messages could still get through.

In the beginning, only government "think tanks" and a few universities were linked. Basically the Internet was an emergency military communications system operated by the Department of Defense's Advanced Research Project Agency (ARPA). The whole operation was referred to as ARPANET.

In time, ARPANET computers were installed at every university in the United States that had defense-related funding. Gradually, the Internet had gone from a military pipeline to a communications tool for scientists. As more scholars came online, the administration of the system transferred from ARPA to the National Science Foundation.

Years later, businesses began using the Internet and the administrative responsibilities were once again transferred.

At this time no one party "operates" the Internet, there are several entities that "oversee" the system and the protocols that are involved.

The speed of the Internet has changed the way people receive information. It combines the immediacy of broadcast with the in-depth coverage of newspapers...making it a perfect source for news and weather information.

Internet usage is at an all time high.

EVOLUTION OF THE INTERNET

Agency (ARPA) funded a research project that created a packet switching network known as the ARPANET. ARPA also funded research projects that produced two satellite networks. In the 1970s ARPA was faced with a dilemma: Each of its networks had advantages for some situations, but each network was incompatible with the others. ARPA focused research on ways that networks could be interconnected and the Internet was envisioned and created to be an interconnection of networks that use TCP/IP protocols. In the early 1980s a group of academic computer scientists formed the Computer Science NETwork, which used TCP/IP protocols.

In the 1980s, as large commercial companies began to use TCP/IP (a protocol, beyond the scope of this book) to build private internets, ARPA investigated transmission of multimedia — audio, video and graphics — across the Internet. Other groups investigated hypertext and created tools such as Gopher that allowed users to browse menus, which are lists of possible options. In 1989 many of these technologies were combined to create the World Wide Web. Initially designed to aid communication among physicists who worked in widely separated locations, the Web became immensely popular and eventually replaced other tools. Also during the late 1980s, the US government began to lift restrictions on who could use the Internet and commercialization of the Internet began. In the early 1990s, with users no longer restricted to the scientific or military communities, the Internet quickly expanded to include universities, companies of all sizes, libraries, public and private schools, local and state governments, individuals and families.

TYPES OF TELECOMMUNICATION NETWORKS

What is a Network?

A network consists of two or more computers that are linked in order to share resources (such as printers and CD-ROMs), exchange files or allow electronic communications. The computers on a network may be linked through cables, telephone lines, radio waves, satellites or infrared light beams.

The basic types of networks include:

- Local Area Network (LAN)
- Wide Area Network (WAN).

LOCAL AREA NETWORK

Local Area Network, in computer science, refers to a collection of interconnected computers that can share data, applications and resources, such as printers. A Local Area Network (LAN) is a network that is confined to a relatively small area. It is generally limited to a geographic area such as a writing lab, school or building. Computers in a LAN are separated by distances of upto a few kilometers and are typically used in offices or across university campuses. A LAN enables the fast and effective transfer of information within a group of users and reduces operational.

In a typical LAN configuration, one computer is designated as the file server. It stores all of the software that controls the network, as well as the software that can be shared by the computers attached to the network. Computers connected to the file server are called workstations. The workstations can be less powerful than the file server and they may have additional software on their hard drives. On most LANs, cables are used to connect the network interface cards in each computer.

Local area networks (LANs), which connect computers separated by short distances, such as in an office or a university campus, commonly use bus, star or ring topologies. Wide area networks (WANs), which connect distant equipment across the country or internationally, often use special leased telephone lines as point-to-point links.

Other connected computer resources are wide area networks (WANs) and private branch exchanges (PBXs). WANs are similar to LANs but they connect computers separated by longer distances, typically across the country or internationally and they use specialized and expensive hardware and leased communications services. PBXs provide continuous computer connections for the transfer of specialized data such as telephone transmissions, but they are not ideally suited to send and receive the short bursts of data used by most computer applications.

INTERNAL LAN CONNECTIONS

A LAN usually consists of a collection of computers, but it also may include printers or data storage devices, such as hard drives. The physical connection between LAN devices can be a coaxial cable, pairs of copper wires or optical fiber. Wireless connections also can be made using infrared or radio-frequency transmissions.

A LAN device can send and receive signals from all other devices in the network. Alternatively, each device may be linked to a repeater or hub, specialized equipment that selectively pass information from one device to one or more destinations in the network.

Networks use protocols or rules, to exchange information through a single shared connection. These protocols prevent collisions of data caused by simultaneous transmission between two or more computers. Computers on most LANs use protocols known as Ethernet or Token Ring. An Ethernet-linked computer checks if a shared connection is in use. If not, the computer transmits data. Since computers can sense an idle connection and send data at the same time, transmitting computers continue to monitor their shared connection and stop transmitting if a collision occurs. Token Ring protocols pass a special message called a token through the network. A computer that receives the token is given permission to send a packet of information or, if the computer has no packet to send, it passes the token to the next computer.

EXTERNAL LAN CONNECTIONS

Connections that link LANs to external resources, such as other LANs or remote databases, are called bridges, routers and gateways. A bridge creates an extended LAN by passing information between two or more LANs. A router is an intermediary device that connects a LAN to a larger LAN or to a WAN by interpreting protocol information and selectively forwarding packets to different LAN or

WAN connections through the most efficient route available. A gateway connects and translates between networks that use different communications protocols. LAN computers use a gateway or router to connect to a WAN such as the Internet, the worldwide consortium of computer networks. Such connections are a security risk because the LAN has no control over users on the Internet. Applications transferred from the Internet to the LAN may contain computer viruses that can harm the components of the LAN or external and unauthorized users may gain access to sensitive files or erase or alter files. A special type of gateway called a firewall keeps external users from accessing resources on the LAN while letting LAN users access the external information.

ADVANCES

Progress in how a network routes information will allow data to move directly from a source computer to a destination computer without interference from other computers. This will enhance the transmission of continuous streams of data, such as audio and video. The wide use of notebook and other portable computers has produced advances in wireless networks. Wireless networks use infrared or radio-frequency transmissions to connect mobile computers to networks. Infrared wireless LANs connect computers within a room, while wireless radio-frequency LANs can connect computers separated by walls.

New LAN technologies will be faster and will support multimedia applications. Asynchronous Transfer Mode (ATM) and Ethernet LANs that are 10 to 15 times faster than standard LANs are now available. To take advantage of faster LANs, computers must become faster, especially the connection called the bus that links the computer's memory to the network. In addition, computer software must be developed that is able to efficiently transfer large amounts of data from networks to computer applications.

WIDE AREA NETWORK

Wide Area Networks (WANs) connect larger geographic areas, such as Florida, the United States or the world. Dedicated transoceanic cabling or satellite uplinks may be used to connect various networks. The following sections discuss the physical topologies used in networks and other related topics:

The physical topology of a network refers to the configuration of cables, computers and other peripherals. Physical topology should not be confused with logical topology which is the method used to pass information between workstations.

Using a WAN, schools in Florida can communicate with places like Tokyo in a matter of minutes, without paying enormous phone bills. A WAN is complicated. It uses multiplexers to connect local and metropolitan networks to global communications networks like the Internet. To users, however, a WAN will not appear to be much different than a LAN or a MAN.

NETWORK TOPOLOGIES

What is a Topology?

The physical topology of a network refers to the configuration of cables, computers and other peripherals. Physical topology should not be confused with logical topology which is the method used to pass information between workstations.

Main Types of Physical Topologies

The following sections discuss the physical topologies used in networks and other related topics:

- Linear bus
- Star
- Star-wired ring
- Tree
- Considerations when choosing a topology.

Linear Bus

A linear bus topology consists of a main run of cable with a terminator at each end (Refer to **Fig. 8.1**). All nodes (file server, workstations and peripherals) are connected to the linear cable. Ethernet and LocalTalk networks use a linear bus topology.

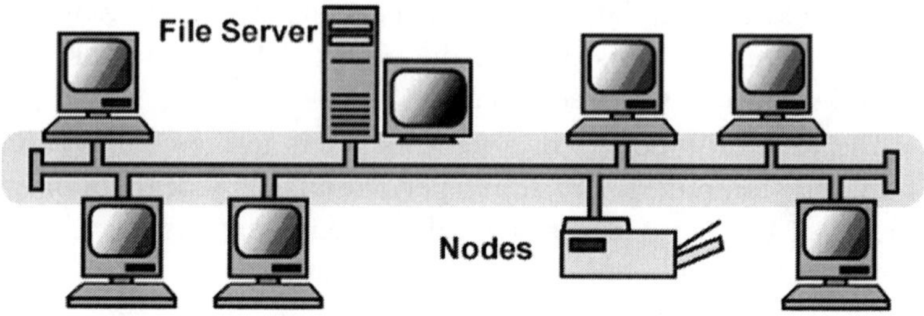

Fig. 8.1: Linear bus topology

Advantages of a Linear Bus Topology

- Easy to connect a computer or peripheral to a linear bus.
- Requires less cable length than a star topology.

Disadvantages of a Linear Bus Topology

- Entire network shuts down if there is a break in the main cable.
- Terminators are required at both ends of the backbone cable.
- Difficult to identify the problem if the entire network shuts down.
- Not meant to be used as a stand-alone solution in a large building.

Star

A star topology is designed with each *node* (file server, workstations and peripherals) connected directly to a central network hub or *concentrator* (Refer to **Fig. 8.2**).

Data on a star network passes through the hub or concentrator before continuing to its destination. The hub or concentrator manages and controls all functions of the network. It also acts as a repeater for the data flow. This configuration is common with twisted pair cable; however, it can also be used with coaxial cable or fiber optic cable.

Advantages of a Star Topology

- Easy to install and wire.
- No disruptions to the network then connecting or removing devices.
- Easy to detect faults and to remove parts.

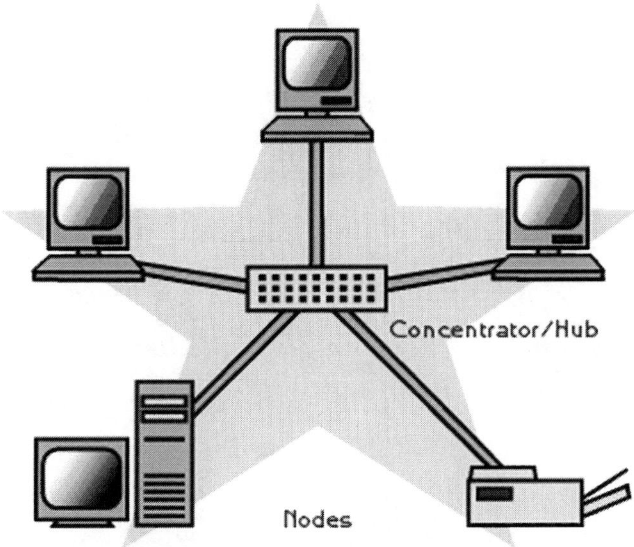

Fig. 8.2: Star topology

Disadvantages of a Star Topology

- Requires more cable length than a linear topology.
- If the hub or concentrator fails, nodes attached are disabled.
- More expensive than linear bus topologies because of the cost of the concentrators.

The protocols used with star configurations are usually Ethernet or LocalTalk. Token ring uses a similar topology, called the star-wired ring.

Star-wired Ring

A star-wired ring topology may appear (externally) to be the same as a star topology. Internally, the **MAU** (multistation access unit) of a star-wired ring contains wiring that allows information to pass from one device to another in a circle or ring. The **Token ring** protocol uses a star-wired ring topology.

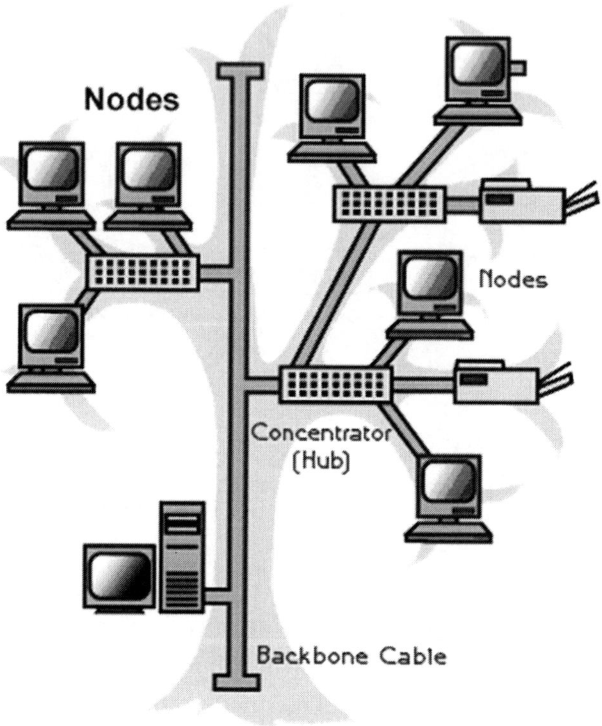

Fig. 8.3: Tree topology

Tree

A tree topology combines characteristics of linear bus and star topologies. It consists of groups of star-configured workstations connected to a linear bus backbone cable (Refer to **Fig. 8.3**). Tree topologies allow for the expansion of an existing network and enable schools to configure a network to meet their needs.

Advantages of a Tree Topology

- Point-to-point wiring for individual segments.
- Supported by several hardware and software venders.

Disadvantages of a Tree Topology

- Overall length of each segment is limited by the type of cabling used.

- If the backbone line breaks, the entire segment goes down.
- More difficult to configure and wire than other topologies.

5-4-3 Rule (For Advanced Knowledge)

A consideration in setting up a tree topology using Ethernet protocol is the 5-4-3 rule. One aspect of the Ethernet protocol requires that a signal sent out on the network cable reach every part of the network within a specified length of time. Each concentrator or repeater that a signal goes through adds a small amount of time. This leads to the rule that between any two nodes on the network there can only be a maximum of 5 segments, connected through 4 repeaters/concentrators. In addition, only 3 of the segments may be populated (trunk) segments if they are made of coaxial cable. A populated segment is one which has one or more nodes attached to it. In **Figure 8.4**, the 5-4-3 rule is adhered to. The furthest two nodes on the network have 4 segments and 3 repeaters/ concentrators between them.

This rule does not apply to other network protocols or Ethernet networks where all fiber optic cabling or a combination of a fiber backbone with UTP cabling is used. If there is a combination of fiber optic backbone and UTP cabling, the rule is simply translated to 7-6-5 rule.

Considerations when Choosing a Topology

- **Money:** A linear bus network may be the least expensive way to install a network; you do not have to purchase concentrators.
- **Length of cable needed:** The linear bus network uses shorter lengths of cable.
- **Future growth:** With a star topology, expanding a network is easily done by adding another concentrator.
- **Cable type:** The most common cable in schools is unshielded twisted pair, which is most often used with star topologies.

Physical Topology	Common Cable	Common Protocol
Linear bus	Twisted pair coaxial fiber	Ethernet localtalk
Star	Twisted pair fiber	Ethernet localtalk
Star-wired ring	Twisted pair	Token ring
Tree	Twisted pair coaxial fiber	Ethernet

Fig. 8.4: Summary chart

SERVICES

Email — How it works

E-mail, in computer science, abbreviation of the term electronic mail, method of transmitting data or text files from one computer to another over an intranet or the Internet. E-mail enables computer users to send messages and data quickly through a local area network or beyond through a nationwide or worldwide communication network. E-mail came into widespread use in the 1990s and has become a major development in business and personal communications.

E-mail users create and send messages from individual computers using commercial e-mail programs or mail-user agents (MUAs). Most of these programs have a text editor for composing messages. The user sends a message to one or more recipients by specifying destination addresses. When a user sends an e-mail message to several recipients at once, it is sometimes called broadcasting.

The address of an e-mail message includes the source and destination of the message. Different addressing conventions are used depending upon the e-mail destination. An interoffice message distributed over an intranet or internal computer network, may have a simple scheme, such as the employee's name, for the e-mail address. E-mail messages sent outside of an intranet are addressed according to the following convention: The first part of the address contains the user's name, followed by the symbol @, the domain name, the institution's or organization's name and finally the country name.

A typical e-mail address might be sally@abc.com. In this example sally is the user's name, abc is the domain name — the specific company organization or institution that the e-mail message is sent to or from and the suffix com indicates the type of organization that abc belongs to — com for commercial org for organization, edu for educational, mil for military and gov for governmental. An e-mail message that originates outside the United States or is sent from the United States to other countries has a supplementary suffix that indicates the country of origin or destination. Examples include uk for the United Kingdom, fr for France and au for Australia.

E-mail data travels from the sender's computer to a network tool called a message transfer agent (MTA) that, depending on the address, either delivers the message within that network of computers or sends it to another MTA for distribution over the Internet. The data file is eventually delivered to the private mailbox of the recipient, who retrieves and reads it using an e-mail program or MUA. The recipient may delete the message, store it, reply to it or forward it to others.

Modems are important devices that have allowed for the use of e-mail beyond local area networks. Modems convert a computer's binary language into an analog signal and transmit the signal over ordinary telephone lines. Modems may be used to send e-mail messages to any destination in the world that has modems and computers able to receive messages.

E-mail messages display technical information called headers and footers above and below the main message body. In part, headers and footers record the sender's and recipient's names and e-mail addresses, the times and dates of message transmission and receipt and the subject of the message.

In addition to the plain text contained in the body of regular e-mail messages, an increasing number of e-mail programs allow the user to send separate files attached to e-mail transmissions. This allows the user to append large text- or graphics-based files to e-mail messages.

E-mail has had a great impact on the amount of information sent worldwide. It has become an important method of transmitting information previously relayed via regular mail, telephone, courier, fax, television and radio.

WWW

World Wide Web (WWW), computer-based network of information resources that combines text and multimedia. The information on the World Wide Web can be accessed and searched through the Internet, a global computer network. The World Wide Web is often referred to simply as "the Web".

Internet topology, the Internet and the Web are each a series of interconnected computer networks. Personal computers or workstations are connected to a Local Area Network (LAN) either by a dial-up connection through a modem and standard phone line or by being directly wired into the LAN. Bridges and hubs link multiple networks to each other. Routers transmit data through networks and determine the best path of transmission.

The Web started to become a popular resource after 1993 when the first widely distributed browser provided a convenient way to access a variety of information on the Internet. The Web uses multimedia, which means that information can be displayed in a wide variety of formats. Users can read text, view pictures, watch animation, listen to sounds and even explore interactive virtual environments on the Web. A user can move seamlessly from a document or Web page stored on the computer to a document or Web page stored on another computer.

The Web offers a place where companies, universities and other institutions and individuals can display information about their products, services, facilities or research or their private lives. Only a small percentage of information on the Web is restricted to subscribers or other authorized users. The majority of Web pages are available to anyone who can access a computer that connects to the Internet. The Web has become a marketplace for many companies selling products or services and a forum for people to exchange opinions and information. Museums, libraries, government agencies and schools post information on the Web to make it available to others.

A WEB OF COMPUTERS

Browser

A browser is a program, such as Microsoft Corporation's Internet Explorer, that allows a computer to display documents containing text, graphics, photographs, sounds, videos and animations. Most browsers are used to view information on the World Wide Web or on intranets of companies or organizations. Browsers have various buttons that allow users to print out the contents of a Web site, move backward or forward between sites already accessed and use a search engine to find information.

All communication on the Web is carried out among a set of computers that are interconnected by a computer network. Web technology can be used across an intranet (a network within a company or organization) or across the global Internet. As with all communications among computers, computers that comprise the Web employ two types of software: client and server. To make information available, a computer runs a server program. To obtain and display information from a server, a computer user runs a client program. The client contacts a server to request information; the server responds by sending a copy of the requested information. To ensure that the exchange is meaningful, the client and server programs must follow a communication protocol, a set of rules that the two programs use to talk to one another. Like a language, a protocol specifies both the form and meaning of each possible message.

In principle, any computer can run a client or a server. In practice, however, large, powerful computers are usually chosen to run server software and small personal computers (PCs) are sufficient to run client software. Powerful computers are chosen for server software because they must be able to handle requests for information from millions of people and do so quickly so that users who request information from the server will not experience long delays. PCs, however, are used by a single person to request a Web page. After a user makes a request, the user waits for the information to be displayed. Thus, the client program running on a user's computer only needs to handle one activity at a time. A server, however, must handle simultaneous requests from many clients, possibly millions.

The difference between the Web and the Internet is similar to the difference between a trucking service and a highway system. The Internet corresponds to a highway that allows traffic to flow between computers and the Web corresponds to a service that uses the highway to move information from one computer to another. Confusion about the difference between the Web and the Internet has arisen because the Web has become extremely popular and currently accounts for the majority of Internet traffic. However, other services also use the Internet to carry their traffic. For example, the Internet's electronic mail service permits users to send and receive textual messages and the file transfer service allows a user to transfer a copy of a file from one computer to another.

Although many services use the Internet to carry data from one computer to another, each service follows a separate set of rules that define the messages used in the exchange. The Web uses the HyperText Transfer Protocol (HTTP, described later in this Chapter), electronic mail uses the Simple Mail Transfer Protocol (SMTP) and file transfer uses the File Transfer Protocol (FTP). The application programs that users run to access the Internet often blur the distinction among these services. For example, an application program that can send e-mail also allows a user to transfer the contents of a file and an application program used to access the Web also allows the user to process e-mail.

HOW THE WEB WORKS?

To access the Web, a user must have a computer connected to the Internet and appropriate software. The connection between the user's computer and the Internet can consist of a permanent, dedicated connection or a temporary, dial-up connection. A dial-up connection uses a modem to send data over the telephone system to another modem. It offers the lowest cost but requires the user to wait for the connection to be established each time the modem is used. A permanent connection uses a technology such as Asymmetric Digital Subscriber Line (ADSL, also known as DSL), a cable modem or a dedicated leased circuit. It remains in place and is ready to use at all times. Permanent Internet connections cost more but offer higher capacity — that is, they can send more data at a faster speed.

Hardware requirements:

1. Computer
2. Modem
3. Telephone line, etc.
4. Internet connection.

Two pieces of software are needed to access the Web:

1. Basic communication software that a computer uses to transfer data across the Internet and
2. A Web application program known as a browser that can contact a Web site to obtain and display information.

Basic communication software, which is usually built into the computer's operating system, allows the computer to interact with the Internet. The software follows a set of protocol standards that are collectively known as TCP/IP (Transmission Control Protocol/ Internet Protocol). Because it is built into the computer's operating system, TCP/IP software remains hidden from users. The software is invoked automatically by application programs that use the Internet.

The second piece of software needed for Web access consists of an application program known as a Web browser. Unlike basic communication software, a browser is directly visible to the user. To access the Web, the user must invoke the browser and enter a request. The browser then acts as a client. The browser contacts a Web server, obtains the requested information and displays the information for the user.

Information on the Web is divided into pages, each of which is assigned a short identification string that is known as a Uniform Resource Locator (URL). A URL encodes three pieces of information: the protocol a browser should use to obtain the item, the name of a computer on which the item is located, including its domain name and the name of the item. For example, the URL http://encarta.msn.com/reference specifies that a browser should use the HyperText Transfer Protocol (HTTP…described later in this Chapter) to obtain the page, that the page can be obtained from a server running on computer, "encarta.msn.com," and that the page is named "reference." The ".com" is the domain name, an abbreviation for commercial, signifying that the site is operated by a commercial or for-profit business. Many other domain names exist, including ".edu" for Web sites established by educational institutions and ".org" for nonprofit organizations.

In 2001 many other unique domain names were created. They comprised ".info" for informational sites, ".biz" for businesses, ".name" for individuals to register their name for a Web site or for an e-mail address, ".museum" for museums, ".aero" for the aviation industry, .coop for business cooperatives such as credit unions and electric coops and ".pro" for professionals such as accountants, lawyers and physicians. As of March 2002, all of these domain name suffixes were operational, with the exception of ".pro."

Only the computer name is required in a URL. If the protocol is omitted, a browser assumes "http://" and if the name of an item is omitted, the server chooses a page to send. Thus, the URL encarta.msn.com, which consists only of a computer name, is also valid.

Before it can obtain information, a browser must be given a URL. A user can enter the URL manually or click on a selectable link. In each case, once it has been given a URL, the browser uses the URL to obtain a new page, which it then displays for the user. The URL associated with a selectable link is not usually visible because the browser does not display the URL for the user. Instead, to indicate that an item is selectable, the browser changes the color of the item on the screen and keeps the URL associated with the link hidden. When a user clicks on an item that corresponds to a selectable link, the browser consults the hidden information to find the appropriate URL, which the browser then follows to the selected page. Because a link can point to any page in the Web, the links are known as hyperlinks.

When a browser uses a URL to obtain a page, the information may be in one of many forms, including text, a graphical image, video or audio. Some Web pages are known as active pages because the page contains a miniature computer program called a script or applet (a small application program). When a script or applet arrives, the browser runs the program. For example, a script can make images appear to move on the user's screen or can allow a user to interact with a mouse, keyboard or microphone. Active pages allow users to play games on the Web, search databases or perform virtual scientific experiments. Active pages are also used to generate moving advertisements, such as a banner that keeps changing or a logo that appears to rotate.

The codes that tell the browser on the client computer how to display a Web document correspond to a set of rules called Hypertext Markup Language (HTML). An HTML document consists of text with special instructions called tags, which are inserted to tell the browser how to display the text. The HTML language specifies the exact rules for a document, including the meaning of each tag. Thus, a person who creates an HTML page is responsible for inserting tags that cause the browser to display the page in the desired form. Not all Web pages use HTML. Graphics images are usually encoded using the Graphics Interchange Format (GIF) or Joint Photographic Experts Group (JPEG) standards. Active pages are written in a computer programming language such as ECMA script or Java.

HTTP

HTTP (for HyperText Transfer Protocol) is the primary method used to convey information on the World Wide Web. The original purpose was to provide a way to publish and receive HTML pages. It is the set of rules for exchanging files (text, graphic images, sound, video and other multimedia files) on the World Wide Web. Relative to the TCP/IP suite of protocols (which are the basis for information exchange on the Internet), HTTP is an application protocol.

TELNET

Telnet, protocol or set of procedures, that enables a user of one computer on the Internet to log on to any other computer on the Internet, provided the user has a password for the distant computer or the distant computer provides publicly available files. Telnet is also the name of a computer program that uses those rules to make connections between computers on the Internet. Many computers that provide large electronic databases, like library catalogs, often allow users to telnet into search the databases. Many resources that were once available only through telnet have now become available on the easier-to-use World Wide Web.

GOPHER

Gopher (computer) is a system that enables computer users to find servers and files on the Internet. Developed at the University of Minnesota in 1991, Gopher presents menus and submenus users can select to specify their search. Each Gopher server contains menus for local servers and files and is linked to other Gopher servers; its menus change as the resources available to the system change. There are hundreds of Gopher servers around the world. The system of all Gopher servers is called Gopherspace.

FAQ?

FAQ, in computer communications, is the abbreviation for Frequently Asked Question, either a commonly asked question or a list of such questions and their answers. FAQs are regularly posted by many newsgroups, mailing lists, forums and other online groups whose participants want to avoid answering the same questions over and over again. Newcomers to such groups are expected to read the FAQs before they participate in group discussions. If newcomers post questions about topics addressed in the FAQs, they may receive angry messages called flames.

Computer Jargon

Application: Software designed for a certain use, such as word processing. Also called a program.

Backspace: A key on the computer keyboard that is marked with the word Backspace or an arrow. Pressing backspace erases characters one at a time to the left of the cursor on the screen. Backspace also deletes anything that has been highlighted.

Bit: The smallest piece of information that is recognized by a computer. It represents a 1 or 0 in the binary numbering system.

Bookmark: To mark a document or a specific place in a document for future reference.

Boot: Derived from "boot strap." To start or restart a computer. A cold boot means to start the computer by turning the power switch on. A warm boot or "reboot" is resetting a computer that is already on.

Browser: A software program that lets you access and navigate the Internet with a graphical interface.

Byte: Eight bits of binary information is a byte, which can represent one letter in the alphabet.

CD-ROM: (Compact Disk–Read Only Memory) A hard plastic disk that holds about 650 megabytes of computer data.

Chat Room: A virtual meeting room where computer users can communicate with each other in real time. People from all over the world can come together in a chat room to discuss topics of mutual interest.

Clicking: Pressing the mouse button. This usually refers to the left mouse button. Double-click means to press the left mouse button twice in quick succession. Right-click means to press the right mouse button.

Computer Case: The plastic structure that houses the main electrical components, which include the CPU. Sometimes referred to as the CPU.

Computer Chip: A thin silicon wafer that contains integrated electronic circuits. Chips perform many computer functions including serving as the computer memory.

CPU: The main component of a computer system. The brain of the computer. Processes all instructions and information.

Cursor: A symbol, usually a solid line or blinking underline character or arrow that signifies where on the screen the next entry will occur.

Delete: A key on the computer keyboard that is marked with the word Delete. (There is often more than one delete key on the keyboard.) Pressing delete erases characters one at a time starting to the right of the cursor on the screen. It also deletes anything that has been highlighted.

Desktop: A metaphor for the on-screen computing environment. A computer desktop includes the screen background, icons and windows visible on the computer screen.

Download: To move or copy a document, program or other data from the Internet or other computer to your computer. The opposite of upload.

E-Mail: Messages sent through a computer network, such as the Internet.

FAQ: (Frequently Asked Questions) Compilation of the most commonly asked questions about a certain subject or product.

Floppy Disk: A thin case enclosing a magnetic disk that stores computer data.

Hard Disk: The storage disk inside of the computer that holds the operating system and programs.

Hard Drive: The hardware mechanism that contains the hard disk.

Hardware: The physical components of a computer system. Refers to objects like disk drives, monitors, keyboards and printers.

Home Page: The main page of a Web site.

HTML: (Hypertext Markup Language) The language that is used to create graphic documents for publication on the Web. Documents that are produced with HTML can have graphics, sound and video in addition to text.

HTTP: (Hypertext Transfer Protocol) The protocol used by the World Wide Web that defines how messages are formatted and transmitted.

Hypertext Link: A word that you click on when on the Web to take you to another Web page or site. These links are usually underlined or in a different color.

Icon: A small picture that represents a program, file or command in your computer system. The program (or file or command) is activated by moving the cursor onto the icon and double-clicking or clicking once and then hitting the Enter key.

Internet: A global web of computers that allows individuals to communicate with each other.

ISP: (Internet Service Provider) A company that lets you dial into their computers in order to connect to the Internet for a fee.

Keyboard: An input device used to type programs, instructions and data into the computer. Similar to the keys on a typewriter.

Log On: Before using the Internet or other on-line service, you are required to log on. This usually entails entering your user name and password.

Megabyte (MB): A unit of computer storage roughly equaling one million bytes.

Megahertz (MHz): Unit of measure used to determine the speed of microprocessors. One MHz represents one million cycles per second. This determines how many instructions per second the microprocessor can execute.

Modem: A device that allows computers to communicate over telephone lines. Modems change the computer's digital signal to an analog signal that can be sent over the telephone lines.

Monitor: A television-like screen that shows you what your computer is doing.

Motherboard: The main circuit board of the computer.

Mouse: An input device that lets you control the computer by controlling the location and action of the cursor on the computer screen.

Operating System: A computer program which acts as the link between the computer and the user.

Printer: A printer transfers graphics and text from your computer to paper.

Program: Software designed for a certain use, such as word processing. Also called an application.

RAM: (Random Access Memory) The temporary memory of the computer where programs and information are kept. The contents of this memory are lost when the computer is turned off.

Screen Saver: A software program that runs some sort of animation on the computer screen when it is turned on, but not in use.

Software: The program or instructions that tell the computer what to do.

Toolbar: A strip of icons in a software program that usually are located at the top and/or bottom of the screen.

Upload: To move or copy a document, program or other data from your computer to the Internet or another computer. The opposite of download.

Web Page: A unit of the World Wide Web. Comparable to a page in a book.

Web Site: Usually consists of several Web pages that share a common focus and has a home page.

World Wide Web (WWW): A portion of the Internet that contains text, audio, graphics and video that are linked together and easily searched with browser software.

Zip Disk: A removable disk that holds more information than a floppy.

Zip Drive: A device for storing information on a type of floppy disk which is much higher density than a regular floppy disk.

Index

COMPUTERS, 1

Classification of Computers, 23
- Mainframes, 26
- Microcomputers, 27
- Minicomputer, 27
- Notebook computers, 27
- Palmtop/Handheld Computers, 28
- Personal computers, 27
- Super computer, 26

Computer Basics, 3
Computers – Working and Related Terms, 4
Disk Drives, 6
Evolution of computers, 13
Exploring Computers, 11
- External or Auxiliary Storage, 11
- Hardware and Software, 11
- Microchips, 12

Generations of Computers, 14
- Fifth Generation, 22
- First Generation: 1946-1958, 15
- Fourth Generation: 1971- Present, 20
- Second Generation: 1959-1964, 17
- Third Generation: 1965-1970, 19
- Zeroth Generation, 14

Hard disk (drive) or HD, 9
Input, 10
Memory, 4
Output, 10
Processing, 8
Storage Devices, 6

DATABASE, 53

Data Abstraction, 58
- Conceptual Level, 59
- Physical Level, 58
- View Level, 59

Data Definition Language (DDL), 65
Data Dictionary, 68
Data Independence, 64
Data Manipulation Language (DML), 65
Data Models, 59
Data, 56
Database Administrator, 66
Database Management Systems, 56
Database Manager, 65
Database Users, 67
Database, 53
Field Types and Widths, 55
Information and its processing, 56
Introduction, 53

Object-based Logical Models, 60
Record-based Logical Model, 62
The E-R Model, 60
The Hierarchical Model, 63
The Network Model, 63
The Object-Oriented Model, 61
The Relational Model, 62
Overall System Structure, 68
Purpose of Database Systems, 57

EXCEL, 108

Automatic Calculation, 131
Setting Automatic Calculation, 131
Trying Automatic Calculation, 131
Changing Font, Font Size, and Font Color, 125
Changing a Single Column Width, 126
Changing the Font Color, 126
Changing the Font Size, 126
Changing the Font, 125
Closing Microsoft Excel, 145
Creating Charts, 140
Change the angle of the data labels, 144
Change the chart scale, 144
Changing Size and Position of Chart, 142
Creating Column Chart, 140
Modify Chart, 143
Deleting Columns, 132
Deleting Rows, 133
Inserting Columns, 133
Inserting Rows, 133
Entering Data, 116
Deleting a Cell Entry, 118
Editing a Cell, 117
Wrapping Text, 118
Entering Text and Numbers, 109
Microsoft Excel Window, 109
Formatting Text and Performing Mathematical Calculations, 119
Adding Bold by Using the Menu, 122
Adding Bold, Underline, and Italic, 122
Adding Italic by Using the Menu, 123
Adding Underline by Using the Menu, 123
Adjusting the Standard Column Width, 119
Cell Alignment, 120
Centering by Using the Menu, 120
Centering by Using the Toolbar, 121
Choosing a Default Font, 119
Left-Aligning by Using the Menu, 121
Left-Aligning by Using the Toolbar, 122

Right-Aligning by Using the Menu, 120
Right-Aligning by Using the Toolbar, 122

Introduction, 108

Moving Quickly Around the Worksheet, 113

Go to — Ctrl-G, 114
Go to — F5, 113
Name Box, 114

Moving to a New Worksheet, 127

MS-Excel Screen, 109

Down Arrow Key, 113
Formula Bar, 111
Menu Bar, 109
Right and Left Arrow Keys, 113
Status Bar, 112
Tab Key, 113
Title Bar, 109
Toolbars, 110
Up Arrow Key, 113
Worksheets, 111

Numbers and Mathematical Calculations, 134

Calculating an Average by Using the Sum Icon, 136
Calculating an Average, 136
Calculating Count, 137
Calculating Maximum, 136
Calculating Minimum, 136
Filling Cells Automatically, 137
Functions, 134
Printing, 139
Reference Operators, 134
Typing a Function, 135

Performing Mathematical Calculations, 128

Addition, 128
AutoSum Icon, 131
Division, 130
Multiplication, 130
Subtraction, 129

Saving File, 145

Selecting Cells, 115

INTERNET, 164

5-4-3 Rule, 173

Advances, 168

Browser, 177

Email, 174

Evolution of the Internet, 165

FAQ, 182

GOPHER, 182

HTTP, 181

Introduction to Internet, 164

Linear Bus, 169

Local Area Network, 166

External LAN connections, 167
Internal LAN connections, 167

Network Topologies, 169

Network, 165

Services, 174

Star, 170

Star-Wired Ring, 171

TELNET, 182

Tree, 172

Telecommunication Networks, 165
Types of Physical Topologies, 169
Wide Area Network, 168
WWW, 176

OPERATING SYSTEM, 29

Autoexec.bat, 41
Basic Commands, 41
Basic DOS structure, 38
Characteristics, 35
Classification, 33
Components, 31
Definition, 29
DOS, 37
File system, 39
Functions & Services, 31
Introduction, 29
MS-DOS, 37
Multiple users, 33
Multi-tasking operating system, 35
Operating System Interfaces, 31
Operating system utilities, 31
Parts, 31
Popular OS, 37
Real-time executive, 32
Single user, 33
Types, 33
Windows, 37

POWERPOINT, 146

First Presentation, 156
Create a Hierarchy, 157
Create a Title Slide, 157
Design Template, 159
Insert a New Slide, 157
Outline and Slides Tab, 159
Print Your Outline, 161
Print Your Slides as a Handout, 163
Print Your Slides, 162
Run Your Slide Show, 161
Slide Sorter View, 161
Use Two-Column Text, 158
Introduction, 146
PowerPoint Overview, 150
Apply a Design Template, 152
Change Your Slides, 152
Correct Spelling, 153
Create New Slides, 150
Print Your Slides, 154
Run Show, 153
Sorter View, 153
PowerPoint Screen, 147
Close Button, 150
Common Tasks Buttons, 149
Drawing Toolbar, 149
Maximize/Restore Button, 150
Menu Bar, 147
Minimize Button, 150
Outline Tab, 148
Placeholders, 148
Rulers, 148
Slides Tab, 148
Standard and Formatting Toolbars, 147
Status Bar, 148

Task Pane, 150
Title Bar, 147
Vertical Splitter Bar, 150
View Buttons, 148
Starting Microsoft PowerPoint, 146

WINDOWS, 70

Clicking, 73
Double Clicking, 75
Dragging, 75
Maximize a Window, 75
Minimize a Window, 75
Configuration, 77
Control Panel, 77
Exploring File Directories, 82
Finding Files on Your Computer, 83
Locating Your Most Recent Files, 83
Opening a Program, 83
File Management, 79
Microsoft Windows, 70
Restarting Windows, 84
Shutting Down Windows, 83
Shutting Down Windows XP, 84
Starting Microsoft Windows, 71
Using the Mouse, 73
Window Desktop, 72
Windows Explorer, 80
Copying from a floppy disk to other drive, 82
Copying file/folder to a floppy disk, 82
Creating Folder, 81
Deleting file or folder, 82
Moving/Copying files to different folders, 82
Renaming File or Folder, 82

WORD PROCESSING & MS WORD, 85

Copying and Pasting, 91
Cutting and Pasting, 93
Entering Text, 87
Formatting Text, 99
Bullets and Numbering, 102
Help, 107
Introduction, 85
Opening and Saving Shortcuts, 105
New File, 105
Opening a File, 106
Saving a File, 106
Opening Your Document, 91
Printing, 96
Print Preview, 96
Re-do 98
Saving a Document, 88
Scroll bars, 104
Spell Checking, 95
Starting and Quitting, 86
Quitting Word, 86
Starting Word, 86
Un-do, 98